ANDREW WEIL, M.D.

Healthy Aging

Andrew Weil, M.D., has devoted the past thirty years to developing, practicing, and teaching others about the principles of integrative medicine. Dr. Weil combines a Harvard education and a lifetime of practicing natural and preventive medicine to provide a unique approach to health care, which encompasses body, mind, and spirit.

He is the Founder and Director of the Program in Integrative Medicine (PIM) at the College of Medicine, University of Arizona, where he is also a Clinical Professor of Medicine and Professor of Public Health and the Lovell-Jones Professor of Integrative Rheumatology. Dr. Weil received both his medical degree and his undergraduate degree in biology (botany) from Harvard University.

PIM, established in 1994, trains physicians, medical students, nurse practitioners, pharmacists, and allied health professionals on the philosophy and practice of integrative medicine. The program's overriding mission is to lead the transformation of medicine and health care throughout the world by creating, educating, and actively supporting a community of professionals who embody the philosophy and practice of integrative medicine.

A world-renowned leader and pioneer in the field of integrative medicine, Dr. Weil is a bestselling author and editorial director of DrWeil.com, the leading online resource for healthy living based on the philosophy of integrative medicine. Dr. Weil's books include the international bestsellers *Spontaneous Healing, Eight Weeks to Optimum Health*, *Eating Well for Optimum Health*, and *The Healthy Kitchen*. He also authors the popular *Self Healing* newsletter and is the Director of Integrative Health & Healing at Miraval Life in Balance Resort. Dr. Weil is an internationally recognized expert on integrative medicine, medicinal plants, mind-body interactions, and the future of medicine and health care. More of his work on aging can be found at www.healthyaging.com. He lives in Arizona.

HEALTHY AGING

HEALTHY AGING

A Lifelong Guide to
Your Well-Being

ANDREW WEIL, M.D.

ANCHOR BOOKS
A Division of Random House, Inc.
New York

FIRST ANCHOR BOOKS EDITION, JANUARY 2007

Copyright © 2005 by Andrew Weil

All rights reserved. Published in the United States by Anchor Books,
a division of Random House, Inc., New York, and in Canada by
Random House of Canada Limited, Toronto. Originally
published in hardcover in the United States by Alfred A. Knopf,
a division of Random House, Inc., New York, in 2005.

Anchor Books and colophon are registered
trademarks of Random House, Inc.

Owing to space limitations, permissions credits
can be found following the index.

The Library of Congress has cataloged the Knopf edition as follows:
Weil, Andrew.
Healthy aging : a lifelong guide to your physical and spiritual well-being /
Andrew Weil.— 1st Knopf ed.
p. cm.
Simultaneously published in Spanish by Vintage Español, a division of
Random House, and in Large Print by Random House.
Includes bibliographical references and index.
1. Aging.   2. Older people—Health and hygiene.   I. Title.
QP86.W445 2005
612.6'7—dc22   2005045183

Anchor ISBN: 978-0-307-27754-1

Book design by Anthea Lingeman

www.anchorbooks.com

Printed in the United States of America
10 9 8 7 6 5 4 3 2 1

Contents

HEALTHY AGING

Introduction

In 2002, I turned sixty. To help celebrate the occasion, friends organized a surprise party for me. After the festivities, there came a time to reflect, and when I did I came to an uncomfortable conclusion: I am closer to a time when my energy and powers will diminish, when I will lose my independence. Sixty is about the time that organs of the body begin gradually to fail, when the first hints of age-related disease begin to appear.

I hardly notice my aging on a day-to-day basis. When I look in the mirror in the morning, my face and white beard seem the same as the day before. But in photographs of myself from the 1970s, my beard is completely black. Looking at old photographs, I can't help but notice the physical change that has taken place in the course of thirty years. If I pay attention, I can notice other changes in my body: more aches and pains, less resilience in meeting the challenges of traveling, less vigor on occasion. And my memory may not be quite what it used to be. At the same time, despite the evidence, some part of me feels unchanged, in fact feels the same as when I was six. Almost everyone I talk to about aging reports similar experiences.

Some years ago I went to my twenty-fifth high school

reunion, the only school reunion I have ever attended. I had not seen most of my classmates since our graduation in 1959. A few of them were just as I remembered them, hardly changed at all, closely matching the images in my memory from a quarter century earlier. Others looked so aged that I could barely find points of coincidence with the pictures of them I had in my head. Why the difference? Why are some individuals so outwardly altered by time and others not? Or, in other words, why is there often a discrepancy between chronological age and biological age? I believe that the answer has to do with complex interactions of genetics and environment. I also believe, based on evidence I have reviewed, that we have control over some of those factors.

I do not subscribe to the view that aging suddenly overtakes us at some point in life, whether at sixty or some other milestone. I meet researchers, physicians, and others who believe that we are born, grow rapidly to maturity, and then coast along on a more or less comfortable plateau until we begin to decline. They call the period of decline *senescence* and consider it distinct and apart from what came before. If one looks only at the physical aspects of life, especially on the cellular level, this is a plausible view.

Cells from old organisms are different from cells of young ones, and observations about how they differ are the basis of biogerontology, the new science of the biology of aging. It is biogerontologists who promote the idea that aging is a programmed phase of decline following the plateau of maturity. In their view senescence is a discrete phase of cellular life coincident with loss of the cells' ability to divide. Senescent cells can still perform many of the functions of life, but they cannot reproduce. When researchers attempt to take cells from organisms, whether plants or animals, and grow them in test tubes, senescence soon overtakes the cultures, cells stop dividing, and the cultures die. (In human life, senescence equates with the period of functional decline that precedes death, with the appearance of age-related diseases.)

By contrast, when cells turn malignant, they often become immune to senescence. Cell biologists refer to this change as *immortalization.* It is one of the most curious and important characteristics of cancer, and I will describe it in more detail later. It points to an equally curious and important possibility about aging, namely, that the mechanics of aging in cells may have evolved as defenses against cancer. Malignant growth may be immortal at the cellular level, but it has the potential to disable and kill entire organisms prematurely—that is, before they can pass on their genes and contribute to the survival and evolution of the species. For life to continue, prevention of malignant growth must be a priority.

In any case, I find it more useful to think of aging as a continuous and necessary process of change that begins with conception. In the words of an Eastern philosopher:

> *The sun at noon is the sun declining;*
> *The person born is the person dying.*

Wherever you are on the continuum of aging, it is important to learn about how to live in appropriate ways in order to maximize health and happiness. That should be an essential goal for all of us. What is appropriate when you are in your twenties is likely not to be appropriate when you are in your fifties.

But I also want to say at the start that I do not believe aging to be reversible. In taking that position, I realize I am taking a risk with those who want to hear that aging *is* reversible, that we will all get to age magnificently. I could say those things, but I won't. If you want to read them, go into any bookstore and you will find no end of titles that are variations on those themes.

The hard fact is that aging will bring unpleasant changes, among them, aches and pains; decreased vigor, healing ability, sensory acuity, muscle tone, bone density, and sexual energy; memory deficits; wrinkles; loss of beauty, friends, family, and independence; increased reliance on doctors and pills; and social isolation. We can mask the outward signs of the process or try to keep up old routines in spite of it, but we cannot change the fact that we are all moving toward physical decline and death. The best we can do—and it is a lot—is to accept this inevitability and try to adapt to it, to be in the best health we can at any age. To my mind the denial of aging and the attempt to fight it are counterproductive, a failure to understand and accept an important aspect of our experience. That attitude is a major obstacle to aging gracefully. To age gracefully means to let nature take its course while doing everything in our power to delay the onset of age-related disease, or, in other words, to live as long and as well as possible, then have a rapid decline at the end of life.

There is a great deal of good news to report about aging too. Happily, most of us will not have to age the way our parents and grandparents did. We have access to better medical treatments for age-related diseases and better knowledge about how to prevent them. We eat better food. We have access to dietary supplements with beneficial effects on health, as well as to other products and services that can help us meet the challenges of growing older. We understand the importance of physical activity and the management of stress. As a result, we are already seeing more and more people in their seventies who look and act the way most people used to look and act in their fifties and sixties, and more eighty-year-olds who are still active, healthy, and enjoying life.

Furthermore, I believe that aging brings rewards as well as challenges and losses. In this book I want to direct your attention to areas of our experience where "old" and "good" are synonymous. What is it that moves us in the presence of old trees? Why are old wines and whiskeys valued much more than young ones? What is it about aged cheeses that improves them so much? Why does age benefit some violins? Why are some antiques so valuable? I want you to consider the qualities in these things that age develops, then look for corresponding qualities in people.

Yes, aging can bring frailty and suffering, but it can also bring depth and richness of experience, complexity of being, serenity, wisdom, and its own kind of power and grace. I am not going to tell you that this or that diet, this or that exercise routine, or this or that herb will make you younger. I am going to try to convince you, however, that it is as desirable to accept aging as it is to take any other steps to improve your health throughout your life. To age gracefully requires that we stop denying the fact of aging and learn and practice what we have to do to keep our bodies and minds in good working order through *all* the phases of life.

The first step toward aging gracefully is to look at the process squarely and understand it for what it is.

PART ONE

*The Science and Philosophy
of Healthy Aging*

1

IMMORTALITY

Question: If you could live forever, would you and why?
Answer: I would not live forever, because we should not
live forever, because if we were supposed to live forever,
then we would live forever, but we cannot live forever,
which is why I would not live forever.

—Miss Alabama in the 1994 Miss USA Contest

Our attitudes toward aging and our responses to the
changes in appearance that aging brings are totally colored
by our knowledge that we are moving inexorably toward
death. It is not my intention to write about death or the fear
of dying in this book, but I find it impossible to avoid men-
tioning them as the source of our negative feelings about
aging, which are entirely based in fear.

Some species age more slowly than we do, others more
rapidly. I have lived with dogs for many years and have
watched several canine companions grow up, grow old, and
die. As I write, I am looking at a photograph from several
years ago of two of my Rhodesian ridgebacks on the front
step of my house in southern Arizona. One is a young male,

Jambo, who could not be more than a year old in the photo. He is standing—sleek, handsome, with all the vitality of youth. The other, B.T., must have been fifteen, very old for such a large breed. She is lying down, her face completely white. Soon she was unable to get up. I helped her through her decline but finally had to euthanize her a day before her sixteenth birthday.

Jambo is now eight years old, still in his prime, still sleek, handsome, and vital, with a deep, soulful personality that makes him an ideal companion animal. Most people who meet him comment on how good-looking he is, the perfect combination of strength and beauty. Sometimes if I am reading in bed at night, I invite him to come up and sit beside me for a few minutes. If I rub his chest in a certain way, he looks up toward the ceiling, extending his neck in a posture of noble contentment that I find very appealing. But when he is in this position, I cannot avoid noticing the first white hairs on his otherwise black chin. And whenever I see them, I also cannot avoid noticing that there are more than the last time I looked.

I know from experience that this dusting of white heralds the changes to come, that one day he, too, will be frosted with the white of old age; and when I see those signs of aging on his strong chin, I think about the disappearance of black from my own facial hair, about the unalterable passage of time, the relentless change of physical bodies as we decline. I think about the pain of the loss of previous companions, about separation from beings I love and who love me, about my own fear of the end and the sadness that is never separable from the joy of human experience. And all of this has come from the observation of a few white hairs on the chin of my dog.

We all sense the finiteness of life, and we all fantasize

about living forever. Is it any wonder, then, that we put so much effort into denying the fact of our aging with cosmetics, plastic surgery, and verbal deceits ("You look so much younger!"), and why we are so enthralled by proponents of antiaging medicine who tell us that we can stop or even turn back the clock?

Immortality is an alluring concept, but I wonder how many of us have thought through its meaning and implications, which turn out not to be so simple. If you lived beyond the normal human life span, what would your life be like? I invite you to look at immortality with me through the lens of biology. Apart from framing this discussion of healthy aging, it will give you a chance to become acquainted with the latest findings of scientists who are studying the aging process. All of the practical advice I have to give you in Part Two of this book is based on this scientific evidence* and grounded in a philosophy that rejects immortality and eternal youthfulness as unworthy goals.

A tension between mortality and immortality is played out on all levels of our being, from our cells to our psyches. Understanding it will help you accept the fact of aging and motivate you to learn to do it as gracefully as possible.

Let's start with immortality on the cellular level. Until 1961, researchers believed that, in theory at least, normal cells, taken from the body and grown in laboratories, should be able to grow and divide forever if their needs were met: if they were provided with a constant supply of food and if their waste products were removed. In that year, Leonard

*For the reader's convenience, a glossary of some of the scientific terms I employ appears after the text.

Hayflick and Paul Moorhead at the Wistar Institute in Philadelphia demonstrated that this was not so, that all normal cells have a fixed limit on the number of times they can divide in order to replace themselves. This number is now known as the Hayflick limit. Hayflick, currently a professor of anatomy at the School of Medicine at the University of California, San Francisco, is one of the foremost biogerontologists. His book *How and Why We Age,* first published in 1994, is the best I have found on the subject. I recommend it highly.

It turns out that the Hayflick limit varies from species to species and often correlates with life span. With a Hayflick limit of about 50 cell divisions, humans are the longest-lived mammals. Mice, which live about three years, have a limit of 15 divisions; for chickens, with an average life span of twelve years, the number is about 25. At the extreme of longevity, the Galápagos tortoise, which can live for 175 years, has a Hayflick limit of 110.

HeLa cells, however, can divide indefinitely. They do not senesce. They continue to grow and divide as long as they have nutrients, oxygen, space, and means of getting rid of their wastes. HeLa cells were the first human cells to be successfully cultured outside the body in large numbers. Given their longevity, they revolutionized biological and medical research and quickly established themselves in laboratories around the world. HeLa cells ignore the Hayflick limit for human cells. In a sense, they are immortal.

I was taught that "HeLa" was composed of the initial letters of the name of a woman, Helen Lane, who was said to be the original source of the cells. This turns out not to have been true. The real source was Henrietta Lacks, a poor African-American woman from Baltimore, whose story only came out years after her cells were growing in prodigious numbers everywhere.

Lacks was born to a family of tobacco pickers in Virginia, moved to Baltimore in 1943 at the age of twenty-three, married, and had five children in quick succession. Then, early in 1951, she noticed she had abnormal vaginal bleeding. She went to a clinic at The Johns Hopkins Hospital, where a doctor found an ominous-looking, quarter-sized tumor on her uterine cervix. He biopsied it and sent the tissue sample off for diagnosis. It was malignant. Shortly afterward, Lacks returned to the clinic to begin radium treatments, but before the first one, another tissue sample from the tumor was taken and sent, this time to George Gey, head of tissue culture research at Johns Hopkins.

Gey, with his wife, Margaret, had been trying to find human cells that would grow well outside the body. His greater goal was to study cancer in order to find a cure. Henrietta Lacks's biopsy gave him exactly what he needed. Her cancer cells grew in test tubes as no other cells had ever grown, vigorously and aggressively. Of course, this did not augur well for their donor. Within months, Lacks's tumor had metastasized throughout her body, creating tumors in all her organs until she expired painfully in a racially segregated ward of The Johns Hopkins Hospital on October 4, 1951, eight months after diagnosis. On the same day, George Gey went on national television to announce his breakthrough in cancer research. He held up a vial of Lacks's cells, calling them, for the first time, HeLa cells.

HeLa cells were soon in great demand. The Geys sent vials of them to colleagues, who sent them to other colleagues, and before long Henrietta Lacks's cancerous cells were multiplying in laboratories throughout the world. They made possible the development of the first polio vaccine, were used to study the effects of drugs and radiation, genetic mechanisms, and many diseases, and were even sent off the planet on a space shuttle to see how cultured human cells would grow in zero gravity. If the HeLa cells world-wide were added up, they would total many, many times the weight of the human being in which they originated.

The saga of Henrietta Lacks raises uncomfortable ethical and social questions, because she never gave informed consent for her cells to be used in this way, neither she nor her family was ever compensated for their use (they did not even find out about all this until twenty-four years after the fact), and none of the scientists who worked with HeLa cells ever acknowledged her contribution. But that is another story.

Why can HeLa cells go on living, perhaps forever, when the human being who produced them is long dead and when most cells senesce after a fixed number of divisions? What determines how many times cells from different organisms can divide? The answers are encoded in DNA, our genetic material. DNA is contained in rodlike structures called chromosomes in the nucleus of every cell. When cells are about to divide in order to reproduce and make more tissue, chromosomes have to replicate themselves, so that each daughter cell will have the same genetic information as its parent cell. The DNA spirals that compose the chromosomes uncoil so that the genetic code can be copied to make duplicate strands, but each time this process occurs, something is lost: a piece of the end of each strand.

Chromosomes terminate in a distinctive region of DNA called a *telomere;* the name comes from Greek roots meaning "end bodies." Telomeres have been likened to the plastic tips at the ends of shoelaces, but that is not an accurate simile, because there is no cap. Rather, the telomere is a repeating sequence of six "letters" (amino acids) of DNA code—TTAGGG—that might be translated in English as THEEND. This sequence repeats thousands of times in a young cell. The mechanics of DNA replication are such that a portion of the telomere is lost with each cell division. At the Hayflick limit, the length of remaining telomere is insufficient to allow further duplication of DNA strands to occur without serious genetic mishaps resulting. So there is no more cell division, no more reproductive life. Instead, there is senescence and, eventually, cell death.

The discovery of telomeres and their possible relationship with the maximum life span of organisms has been one of the most important advances in the fields of genetics and biogerontology. It has allowed researchers to solve one of the great mysteries of cancer—namely, how cancer cells become immortal and go on dividing until they kill the organism in which they arise. In 1985, Drs. Carol Greider and Elizabeth Blackburn reported the discovery of telomerase, an enzyme that adds more six-letter units to telomeres, making up for their normal loss during cell division. They first found it in a microscopic one-celled animal called *Tetrahymena* that lives in freshwater lakes and streams and is commonly used in genetics research, but telomerase has since been found in many multicellular organisms, including humans. Although it almost never occurs in normal cells, most cancer cells produce it.

Malignant transformation is a complex process involving the suppression of some genes and the activation of others, sometimes in response to carcinogenic agents, sometimes not. Malignant cells are unresponsive to general controls on growth and development and a threat to their normal neighbors, but it is a long way from malignant transformation of one or many cells to a clinically significant cancer with the potential to kill its host. Many cancer cells die because their genetics and metabolism are hopelessly deranged or because they outgrow their blood supply. Others are weeded out by the body's defensive systems. Those that survive will run up against the Hayflick limit—unless they acquire the ability to produce telomerase. A gene for telomerase expression is present in many cells but is inactive. (I will explain why it's there in a moment.) If a cancer cell manages to turn it on, and thus produce the enzyme to lengthen telomeres, it can divide indefinitely, giving rise to a clone of malignant cells that can eventually become a detectable tumor.

This is what happened in Henrietta Lacks's cervix. HeLa cells owe their unlimited growth to telomerase. Telomerase expression is probably not the only path to cellular immortality, because 10 percent of tumors seem able to rebuild their telomeres without it; evidently, they find some other gene product to achieve the same end. As researchers close in on the fine details of cellular immortalization, new possibilities for cancer diagnosis and treatment may emerge. Detection of telomerase in tissue samples may announce the presence of cancer in its earliest, most curable stages. If we can find a way to suppress telomerase expression—to turn off the gene that controls it—we may be able to render cancer cells mortal again and stop their relentless growth. That may take too long to be a primary treatment, but it may be very useful as a backup approach to prevent metastasis, without the toxicity of conventional chemotherapy.

I said I would explain why the potential to produce telomerase exists in most cells, even though it is not realized. The reason is that some nonmalignant cells need this enzyme and use it in the course of normal growth and development. Examples are embryonic stem cells (which direct the growth of embryos and can be taken from them), adult stem cells (which persist in some tissues of mature organisms), and germ cells (which can create new organisms). I'll save a discussion of germ cells—eggs and sperm—for later. Embryonic stem cells are universal cells that have the potential to grow and differentiate in unlimited ways. They can give rise to any type of cells in an organism, from skin cells to blood cells to nerve cells. (In other words, all cells stem from them.) In general, the more differentiated and specialized cells are, the less is their potential to replicate themselves and change. Heart muscle cells and neurons in the brain are the most specialized cells in the body. They are at the opposite end of the spectrum from embryonic stem cells. Their functions are limited and highly focused, they cannot divide or replace themselves, and when they die they are permanently lost.

Yet both kinds of cells contain the full human genome in their chromosomes. The difference is in which genes are expressed—turned on—and which are not. In stem cells many genes are activated that in mature cells are turned off, among them the gene for expression of telomerase. The work of embryonic stem cells ends with the construction of a new, complete organism. At that point, it is important that their activities cease. They may evolve into adult stem cells, which I describe below, but there is no place for these totipotent, universal powerhouse cells in a developed organism. In fact, if they persist, they may give rise to the fast-growing cancers that appear in children and young adults and that are of different origin from the usual cancers that occur in older people.

Cancers of childhood include retinoblastoma (eye), neuroblastoma (adrenal gland), and Wilms' tumor (kidney). Horrific diseases though they are, they are uniquely susceptible to chemotherapy and radiation because their cell division rates are so high. (Chemotherapy and radiation target dividing cells.) The cancers of childhood are considered to be born of embryonic cells, again emphasizing the close relationship between immortality and malignant growth.

Embryonic stem cells have been much in the news lately as researchers have come to appreciate the possibility of using them to regenerate damaged tissues and organs and treat age-related ailments such as Parkinson's disease. This line of investigation has incurred the wrath of the religious right, which opposes all research involving human embryos and has managed to shut down government funding for work with embryonic stem cells. Privately funded research in this area will certainly continue; federally funded scientists may have to shift their attention to work with adult stem cells, which do not require embryos as a source but are more limited in their potential medical usefulness.

Osteosarcoma, or primary bone cancer, is an example of a cancer that strikes young adults; the typical age of onset is between ten and twenty years. It is probably also of stem cell origin but likely arises from an aberrant adult stem cell. Many but not all adult tissues contain these relatively rare "primitive" cells that have the potential to differentiate into all the cells making up that tissue. For example, stem cells in the bone marrow can not only replicate themselves but also develop into precursors of all the different varieties of white blood cells, red blood cells, and platelet-producing cells. Adult stem cells in connective tissue can give rise to cells of bone, cartilage, muscle, and fat. Adult stem cells are not as universal in their capacities as embryonic stem cells, but they are still marvelously creative. And they still have the negative potential of spawning fast-growing cancers.

At present, doctors perform adult stem-cell transplants to regenerate bone marrow in selected cancer patients, a great improvement over the older method of transplanting marrow itself. (Bone marrow is the source of red blood cells, white blood cells, and platelets.) For some leukemias, lymphomas, and multiple myeloma stem cell transplants can be lifesaving. The method is to harvest these special cells from the bone marrow or from circulating blood, then destroy existing bone marrow (and any malignant cells it harbors) with high-dose chemotherapy, radiation, or both. Ordinarily, this would result in rapid death, but when the stem cells are reinfused into the bloodstream, they go right to the depleted marrow and regenerate all the needed cell lines, all free of disease.*

But this is just the beginning of what stem cells might accomplish. If you do an Internet search on "stem cells," you will get a sense of current and future possibilities. Stem cells might provide cures for diseases that have always been considered incurable (like Alzheimer's disease and juvenile diabetes), restore hearing in cases of nerve deafness, even allow regeneration of damaged spinal cords.

I have written elsewhere:

> Heart muscle that is lost as a result of interruption of blood supply in a heart attack is not replaced by muscle. Healing occurs in the form of a fibrous scar, but there is no regeneration of the original tissue. The same is true of neurons in the brain. Heart muscle cells and nerve cells are so specialized in function—so differentiated— that they seem to have lost the capacity for new growth. Yet perhaps even in these vital cells there are switches waiting to be discovered that might turn on the appropriate sequences of DNA in the nucleus. If science begins

---

*There is another potential source of blood-forming stem cells: the blood in the umbilical cord of a newborn. This blood can be harvested just after birth, frozen, and kept in storage for possible future use by that person or by another person of compatible blood and tissue type. Expectant parents should be encouraged to request this safe procedure.

to focus on the healing system, isolating and understanding its mechanisms . . . it is not impossible that doctors will one day be able to spark the regeneration of damaged hearts and brains and severed spinal cords. That will truly be a new era of healing-oriented medicine.

The key to these wonderful possibilities now appears to be the harnessing and directing of potentially immortal cells that exist in the body both during embryonic development and in maturity. But I must remind readers again of the link between immortality and cancer. One vision of immortality is the rampant growth of HeLa cells that killed their host. Both embryonic and adult stem cells must keep their appointed limits to avoid this kind of disaster. Possibly they express telomerase transiently, during phases of active growth, then turn its production off when rapid growth is no longer appropriate.

There is another line of telomerase research that also raises both hopes and fears. It is now possible to insert the gene for this enzyme into cells that lack it and so enable mature cells to lengthen their telomeres and rejuvenate. This has been successful with human fibroblasts, cells found in the skin that have some of the potential of adult stem cells. Fibroblasts manufacture the elastic fibers and collagen that give tone to the skin, and they can also differentiate along various pathways to produce cells that compose fat, bone, cartilage, and smooth muscle. The senescence of fibroblasts—a consequence of telomere loss—underlies the deterioration of skin with age and may be the cause of age-related changes in other tissues these cells support.

Some evidence for this comes from studies of a rare inherited disease, Werner's syndrome, characterized by accelerated aging, at least of some parts of the body. The symptoms of Werner's syndrome appear in adolescence and include eye cataracts, loss and graying of hair, skin wasting, accelerated osteoporosis and atherosclerosis, and increased suscepti- bility to cancer (probably the result of deterioration of immune function). Those afflicted rarely live beyond their late forties, by which time they look like people twice as old. Their prematurely aged skin is particularly striking. Fibro- blasts taken from the skin of Werner's syndrome patients and cultured in the laboratory show abnormally shortened telomeres and premature senescence. But if the gene for making telomerase is supplied to these ailing fibroblasts in test tubes, they rejuvenate: their telomeres lengthen, the fibroblasts resume all of their functions, and they may even immortalize *without showing signs of malignant transformation*.

This experiment raises several important possibilities. First, it points up the fact that immortalization is not neces- sarily synonymous with cancer, even though it often goes hand in hand with it. Immortalization by way of telomerase is a tool acquired and used, often with dreadful conse- quences to organisms, by cells gone bad. In nonmalignant cells it may lead to rejuvenation with beneficial conse- quences to organisms, as long as production of the enzyme can be controlled—that is, turned on when needed and turned off when not.

Second, the experiment suggests that treatments for the damage caused by Werner's syndrome may be forthcoming, not just for the skin damage but possibly for the more seri- ous problems. For example, it is abnormal fibroblast activity that causes thickening of the smooth muscle in the walls of arteries. This, in turn, narrows the interior of arteries and is one of the changes contributing to atherosclerosis. (Many

Werner's syndrome patients die from their cardiovascular disease.)

Third, there is the possibility of an effective method of rejuvenating skin. For many people the wrinkling, thinning, and sagging of skin with the passage of time are among the most distressing effects of aging, and a cosmetics industry selling billions of dollars of products and services caters to that distress. Many of those products and services are worthless. (I'll discuss them later.) But imagine if skin could really be made young again by supplying it with rejuvenated, immortal fibroblasts, ready and able to nourish it, tighten it up, repair damage, and make it glow. That may be on the horizon. Just imagine the ramifications—medical, cosmetic, and commercial!

Finally, one can glimpse the distant possibility of a more general system of regenerative medicine using genetic manipulation to enable fibroblasts and other basic cell types to repair inborn or acquired damage to many organs and tissues, so that we could effectively and safely treat conditions like pulmonary fibrosis, atherosclerosis, osteoporosis, and degenerative brain diseases. Research with fibroblasts and telomerase hints at a potential aspect of what medicine of the future could be, one that is strikingly beneficial.

Again, however, I want to inject a note of caution and concern. Cellular immortality is fascinating, but I find it disturbing as well, especially when it is invoked as a key to life extension. Let me quote an expert on the subject, Professor S. Jay Olshansky from the School of Public Health at the University of Illinois at Chicago. Olshansky is the coauthor (with Bruce A. Carnes) of *The Quest for Immortality: Science at the Frontiers of Aging,* an excellent book, and also one of the principal authors (the others are Carnes and Hayflick) of the "Position Statement on Human Aging," published in 2002. The intent of the "Position Statement" was to counter many of the claims made by proponents of antiaging medicine; it was signed by dozens of scientists and experts on aging, including me, and received a great deal of publicity. Here is what the statement says about telomeres and longevity:

> Solid scientific evidence has shown that telomere length plays a role in determining cellular life span in normal human fibroblasts and some other normal cell types. However, increasing the number of times a cell can divide may predispose cells to tumor formation. Thus, although telomere shortening may play a role in limiting cellular life span, there is no evidence that telomere shortening plays a role in the determination of human longevity.

The growth of cells in a culture may have little to do with the behavior of cells in the body, and the possibility of rejuvenating fibroblasts with telomerase may tell us little about whether we can manipulate human life span. There is a division of scientific thinking here. Some see telomerase as a modern version of the fountain of youth. Others are skeptical. I will wait and see.

Now I want to look at a third category of potentially immortal cells, those that carry on the function of reproduction. All cells of the body except ova and spermatozoa have duplicate sets of chromosomes, one from each parent. When cells divide asexually, the chromosomes are reproduced in their entirety, and each daughter cell inherits the same duplicate set. But when germ cells—eggs and sperm—form, the sets split, one of each going to each daughter cell. Thus, germ cells have half the number of chromosomes of somatic (body) cells, so that when an egg and sperm fuse, the fertilized egg—and all cells derived from it, except the germ cells of the next generation—will have a genetic set from each parent.

In essence, sexual reproduction is a reshuffling of the genetic deck, so that offspring will have a somewhat different set of inherited characteristics from parents. A few organisms, such as some yeasts, don't bother with sexual reproduction; they just bud off daughter cells with identical genes that go off on their own. But nature has strongly favored the sexual method because it confers great advantages on species, if not on individuals.

In the desert where I live outside of Tucson, Arizona, the most dangerous cactus is the jumping cholla *(Opuntia fulgida),* a relative of the better-known and much less dangerous prickly pear, which is bad enough if you stumble into it. Jumping chollas have round, jointed stems armed with fearsome spines that are marvels of botanical engineering. They are so sharp that they pierce skin and flesh deeply with the slightest pressure, and they are covered with microscopic reverse barbs that make extracting them difficult and painful. Unwary humans—and dogs and other animals—who make contact with this plant often find a whole joint of it embedded in a thigh or arm. This is especially surprising when you are not even aware of contact; it seems as if a whole section of the cactus has jumped from the plant to your flesh. In fact, jumping chollas do not jump, but their spiny, jointed stems break off with the slightest tug. What I think happens is that minimal contact with the plant allows a few spines to pierce the skin, and before this even registers on consciousness, there is a reflex jerk of the extremity, which causes a whole section of stem to detach from the plant and embed itself deeply and firmly.

This is actually a highly successful reproductive strategy of the jumping cholla, because that detached piece of cactus will root itself and grow a new plant as soon as an animal or human gets it out and leaves it on the desert floor. This is "vegetative reproduction"—no genetic reshuffling involved—and is the basis of propagating desirable varieties of plants by cuttings, grafting, and budding rather than by collecting and planting seeds. Vegetative reproduction preserves the genetic characteristics of the plant that provides the somatic tissue. The jumping cholla is very good at this; some tracts of the Sonoran Desert are mainly cholla forests, very difficult to walk through without heavy footwear and a lot of careful stepping. In fact, this species of cactus is so efficient at this means of reproduction that it has lost the ability to reproduce sexually. It makes clusters of seedy fruits like other cholla species, but the seeds are sterile. All of the jumping chollas in this vast desert are clones with identical genetics.

So far, so good. The jumping cholla would seem to be a very successful species. There are certainly plenty of them; they all look healthy; and by "jumping" anything that brushes against them, they reproduce like crazy. Yet they are extremely vulnerable. Genetic variation is nature's chief hedge against environmental change. Should the environment of the Sonoran Desert shift—if it were to become much colder or wetter, for example, or if a new fungal disease that attacked cacti were to appear—the jumping chollas might soon be doomed. The entire population could be wiped out very quickly, and *Opuntia fulgida* would then be relegated to the long list of extinct species that have failed to continue living on planet Earth.

Life here evolved in hostile, changing environments, and there is no reason to believe that things will get any easier. Sex shuffles the genetic deck in order to create a wide variety of possibilities, so that some individuals will survive an environmental cataclysm even if most do not. In this way, the species will go on, although individuals die. Sex is a very successful strategy for the perpetuation of life at the species level, but it exacts a very high price on individuals, namely, death. Any meaningful discussion of immortality must look at this trade-off.

In *The Quest for Immortality,* Olshansky and Carnes write: "It is genes which are immortal, not the bodies that carry them. Genes, the ultimate time travelers, transcend the bounds of time that measures the limits imposed on our mortal bodies." DNA and the genes within it are immortal. They encode instructions for building mortal bodies that serve to perpetuate them. The DNA in your cells is the present chapter in an unbroken lineage that goes back to the first DNA to appear on Earth. Most scientists believe that this self-replicating molecule evolved spontaneously from simple organic compounds that accumulated in water under the very different physical conditions that existed on Earth in the distant past. A dissenting minority believe that our planet was seeded with DNA from elsewhere, that this unique molecule arrived preformed from outer space and proceeded to use the raw materials of Earth to construct mortal bodies for its own purposes.

In any case, the germ cells that carry DNA to the next generation are the vehicles for the immortality of DNA but are not themselves immortal. Ova that are not fertilized die soon after ovulation, and spermatozoa have a short life span. But both types of cells have functioning genes for telomerase, and if these genes are disabled, normal fertilization is impaired. Of course, once fertilization occurs, the resulting zygote depends on telomerase for explosive cell division and growth into an embryo. Moreover, germ cells are special in another way that makes them of great interest to biogerontologists: their DNA repair systems are significantly more efficient than those of somatic cells.

One theory of aging postulates accumulated errors in the DNA of somatic cells as the root cause of degenerative change. From this point of view, the wrinkling of skin, the hardening of arteries, the loss of brain cells, and other characteristics that distinguish old humans from young humans equate with cumulative damage to DNA over time and consequent flaws in the content and translation of genetic instructions in cells. There is no question that DNA is susceptible to damage. Its strands can be broken or deformed by a variety of chemical agents (like free radicals, which I will discuss later) and energetic insults (like ultraviolet rays from the sun, cosmic rays, and X-rays). Accidents in the normal course of DNA replication may also result in genetic garbling. If cell division occurs before repair, the damage is passed on to daughter cells and genetic errors accumulate.

In order to protect against these calamities, DNA contains instructions for the manufacture of enzymes to repair itself and to neutralize potentially damaging agents. Cellular life represents a continual battle between the forces that damage DNA and the mechanisms of DNA repair. Thomas Perls, M.D., who has studied the genetics of longevity at Harvard, says what is remarkable about all of this is how long we live now, given the hostility of the environment and the multiplicity of forces that create errors in DNA. "The wonder is not that we age and die but that we make it through life as well as we do," he says.

If somatic cells need to protect themselves from damage

to DNA, think how much more important that is for germ cells, which must deliver DNA from generation to generation as intact as possible. The mechanisms of DNA repair in germ cells must be in the best operating order at all times. Understanding those mechanisms in germ cells might enable us to boost them in somatic cells and thus approach rejuvenation of tissues and organs in another way, one not dependent on telomerase. This is yet another possibility on the horizon of medicine.

In writing about immortality, I have kept mostly to the cellular level. But what are the possibilities for immortality of the organism? Or, if not immortality, then extended longevity?

Again, I find reasons for caution. A grotesque possibility is depicted in the Greek myth of Tithonus. Eos, goddess of the dawn, has an affair with Ares, the significant other of Aphrodite. To punish Eos, Aphrodite makes her fall in love with beautiful mortals. Eos finds two of them, Tithonus and Ganymede, but the ruler of the gods, Zeus, also wants Ganymede and takes the youth to Olympus to be his cupbearer. Zeus offers to repay Eos for taking Ganymede by promising to fulfill one wish: Eos wishes for Tithonus to be immortal, forgetting to ask that he remain eternally youthful. The result is that Tithonus lives forever but ages relentlessly until he is an ancient, shriveled, suffering creature. Eos shuts him away to spend eternity thus, although in some versions of the story he is changed into a grasshopper or cricket and kept in a cage. (Those insects are symbols of longevity in some cultures.)

Modern medicine is already capable of producing Tithonian outcomes—extending life without preserving health—

and if it gains techniques for dramatically extending the life spans of cells, tissues, and organs, the consequences to organisms could be dismal. Be wary of wishing for life extension without thinking through the details of what your extended life will be like.

Suppose some power could grant your wish for eternal youth and health along with unlimited years. How long could you stand that?

Writers and philosophers throughout history have speculated on the possibility of immortality; almost all have concluded that it would be intolerable. A favorite novel of mine that touches on this theme is *The Sibyl,* written in 1956 by Nobel laureate Pär Lagerkvist, a tale that might be summarized as the Wandering Jew meets a defrocked priestess of the Delphic Oracle. In it, the Jewish character seeks out the priestess in an effort to understand and come to terms with his peculiar fate. He had refused Jesus's request to lean against his house and rest a moment before continuing to drag the cross on his way to be crucified. "I thought, If a condemned man, a man so unhappy, leans against my house, he may bring ill fortune upon it. So I told him to move on, and said I didn't want him there."

"Because I may not lean my head against your house your soul shall be unblessed forever . . ." was Jesus's response. "Because you denied me this, you shall suffer greater punishment than mine: you shall never die. You shall wander through this world to all eternity, and find no rest."

Much later, as the Wandering Jew began to realize the import of these words, this truly unfortunate man glimpsed his future:

It was strange; he had said that I should live forever— that I should never die. How strange. . . . Why should I mind that? Had it not always been my dearest wish never to have to die, never to die? Why then did I not rejoice? Why did I feel no gladness?

. . . "to all eternity, and find no rest."

I had never really thought about it before, but now I seemed to gain some inkling of what eternity was. That it would deprive me of life. That it was itself the damnation, the unblessedness, that it would itself unhallow my soul.

Eternity. . . . It has nothing to do with life, I thought; it is the contrary to all life. It is something limitless, endless, a realm of death which the living must look into with horror. Was it here that I was to dwell? Was it for that that this thing had been given me? "To all eternity. . . ." That was my death sentence: the most cruel that could be devised.

The conclusion of all philosophers and writers who consider immortality is the same as that of Lagerkvist's unhappy character. Aging and death give meaning to life. Without them, life would eventually be horrible, intolerable. We may wish to live longer than the biblical allotment of three score years and ten, or more than the somewhat greater life expectancy of people born today in countries of the industrialized world who enjoy the blessings of modern medicine. Certainly, we may legitimately hope that the diminishments and ravages of old age come late in our lifetimes and that decline and death be swift and peaceful. But to yearn for eternal youth and escape from death seems to me the height of foolishness.

I have held up several different visions of immortality in this chapter, all of which reinforce the conclusion of the writers and philosophers, even if they did not have access to the information being discovered by the biogerontologists of today. The first is the identity of cellular immortality and malignant growth. When cells become immortal, they are cancerous. They disregard the rules that govern the normal growth and development of organisms, behave in ways dangerous and selfish, and ultimately destroy the organisms in which they arise. The second is the sterility of life without sex and death, as illustrated by the jumping cholla and its inability to adapt to a changing environment. The third is the Tithonian disaster: entrapment in the inevitable suffering of life with no possibility of release. A fourth is the fate of the Wandering Jew, robbed by eternal life on Earth of everything that makes real life worth living.

I wanted to present these ideas at the beginning of this book because of the tremendous power that the concept of antiaging exerts over contemporary minds. Antiaging medicine is a major current in contemporary health care, now spawning journals, conventions, clinics, practitioners, and very brisk markets for products and services. Antiaging proponents may not exactly be offering immortality or eternal youth, but they are clearly tapping into widespread human longing for those outcomes. I will examine the antiaging movement in some detail in a succeeding chapter because I feel strongly that it impedes many people from coming to a healthy and positive acceptance of both aging and mortality.

Alfred, Lord Tennyson (1809–92) wrote a poem called "Tithonus." It opens:

> *The woods decay, the woods decay and fall,*
> *The vapours weep their burthen to the ground,*
> *Man comes and tills the field and lies beneath,*

And after many a summer dies the swan.
Me only cruel immortality
Consumes; I wither slowly in thine arms. . . .

Go back and read the words of Miss Alabama that precede this chapter. Perhaps you will find more wisdom in them now than at first reading.

2

SHANGRI-LAS AND FOUNTAINS OF YOUTH

> Never had Shangri-La offered more concentrated loveliness to his eyes; the valley lay imaged over the edge of the cliff, and the image was of a deep unrippled pool that matched the peace of his own thoughts.

—James Hilton, *Lost Horizon* (1933)

In *The Quest for Immortality*, Olshansky and Carnes identify three universal and pervasive categories of legends about living forever and retaining youth. They call these the *antediluvian, hyperborean,* and *fountain* legends.

Antediluvian ("before the flood") fantasies concern some prior age in which people supposedly lived much longer than they do today or lived forever or were eternally young. Hyperborean ("beyond the north wind") legends describe the same things but assign them to remote or magical locales, protected from the corrupting influences of the familiar world. Fountain (i.e., fountain-of-youth) stories describe magical substances that reverse aging and negate death.

There is solid scientific evidence that people today live

longer than people ever have, even that human life span has slowly increased in the course of evolution. There is no scientific evidence for greater longevity in any past age. Biblical claims that Methuselah and others made centenarians look like youngsters are soundly contradicted by the findings of paleontologists.

Nor is there any reason to believe that very long-lived people populate any particular region of the world. (I will, however, look at a few places that seem to me worth studying for clues about healthy aging.)

Fountain legends are not so easy to dismiss. Telomerase and stem cells may be very far from what Ponce de León had in mind when he roamed the West Indies in 1513 in search of Bimini and its magical spring (natives of what is now Puerto Rico told him about it), but today we are working with materials that may have some of its storied rejuvenating properties. This subject deserves closer scrutiny, because it is the theme played by marketers of antiaging products and services.

Before I tackle it, I would like to look briefly at a modern legend of longevity and lasting youth that captured the collective imagination of the world—at least of the Western world—in the middle of the twentieth century. James Hilton's novel *Lost Horizon*, published in 1933, seems to be purely hyperborean in its description of the lamasery of Shangri-La, hidden away in pristine splendor in the Valley of the Blue Moon, somewhere beyond the highest Himalayas. Actually, it is also a fountain story, since the inhabitants attribute their extraordinary health and long life in part to a native plant, a detail often overlooked by commentators. This occurs to Conway, the hero of the novel, shortly after his arrival: "He liked Chinese cooking, with its subtle undertones of taste; and his first meal at Shangri-La had therefore conveyed a welcome familiarity. He suspected, too, that it might have contained some herb or drug to relieve respiration, for he not only felt a difference himself, but could observe a greater ease among his fellow guests." The secret ingredient is later identified as "the *tangatze* berry, to which were ascribed medicinal properties, but which was chiefly popular because its effects were those of a mild narcotic."

Father Perrault, a Capuchin friar and the High Lama of Shangri-La, who combines the most benign aspects of Christianity with those of Buddhism and has lived for several centuries, tells Conway that when he arrived at the lamasery, he "plunged forthwith into rigorous self-discipline somewhat curiously combined with narcotic indulgence," or, in other words, "drug taking and deep-breathing exercises." So the extreme longevity of the inhabitants of this magical paradise is due both to a substance and to isolation from the noxious influences of a world that is toxic on all levels: physical, mental, and spiritual.

Hilton's novel must have had special appeal for the generation about to be engulfed by the Second World War, but it seems to me that the allure of these two possibilities remains timeless and universal. If only we could neutralize the toxic assaults of the world around us, we might avoid or at least mitigate the ravages of time. And there must be remedies we can take to stave off aging and death.

Some years ago, researchers went to several remote regions to try to verify claims of extraordinary longevity. Three of these were Abkhazia in the Caucasus region of the former Soviet Union; Hunzakut, a valley in Pakistan; and Vilcabamba in Ecuador. The only one that I have personal experience of is the last, which did not seem different to me from any of the other Andean Indian villages I visited in Ecuador.

In every case, the claims turned out to be unsubstantiated,

because there were no reliable birth records. In fact, strong evidence turned up that old people in these places exaggerated their ages for various reasons, even that some of them used the birth dates of deceased older siblings. In Abkhazia, investigators uncovered a clear pattern of state-supported falsification of birth records in order to develop unusual longevity as a national resource and tourist attraction.

Before the scientific community reached a consensus about the lack of evidence for these claims, many articles appeared in the popular press about the lifestyles of Abkhazians, Hunzakuts, and Vilcabambans that attempted to find commonalities. Most of the residents of the regions, as one might have expected, were physically active into old age; indeed, their traditional lifestyles demanded it, because they had to herd animals, gather wood, carry water, and till fields. They ate well, eating more fresh foods than typical Westerners and no fast or processed foods. The Abkhazians had frequent feasts, featuring local fruits, vegetables, and meat, as well as yogurt, which is often touted as a magical rejuvenator. They also consumed alcohol at these gatherings. In all of the regions, strong communal ties were evident, and early investigators made much of the contribution of these ties to supposed unusual longevity.

Some of these practices are obvious features of healthy lifestyles and may well increase the probability of aging gracefully. In particular, I think that ongoing physical activity and strong social and communal ties are most important. I am not alone in this. In 1998, John W. Rowe, M.D., and Robert L. Kahn, Ph.D., wrote *Successful Aging,* a summary of the MacArthur Foundation Study of Aging in America, begun in 1987. Sixteen scientists from different fields collaborated on this project, which included studies of over a thousand well-functioning older people. The scientists identified maintenance of physical activity throughout life and maintenance of social and intellectual connectedness as the two outstanding common features of the lifestyles of their subjects. These characteristics were more prominent than any particular dietary patterns or the use of dietary supplements.

Studies of centenarians have become more common as more people throughout the world live to be one hundred. In Japan, America, and Scandinavia, the percentage increase in centenarians in recent years has been dramatic. In fact, in those countries the oldest old constitute the fastest-growing segment of the population. Most centenarians are female, and most are ailing, but some are in remarkably good shape. Are there any commonalities to be discovered in the lifestyles, attitudes, or behavior of the healthy oldest old?

A number of centers for centenarian studies now exist—in Okinawa, Germany, the United States, and other countries. A problem with this kind of research is that criteria for recruiting subjects are often not made clear, raising questions about whether any population samples are representative. It is not easy to conduct studies of centenarians, and those who end up as subjects may be healthier and better functioning than those left out. The only way to correct for such selection bias is to study *all* individuals one hundred years or older in a defined geographical region.

In the United States, centenarian studies have recently been brought under the central coordination of the University of Georgia Gerontology Center and the direction of Leonard W. Poon. Poon points out that there is no such thing as a typical centenarian: "You can't make generalizations about these very exceptional people because each one is different. Centenarians continue to surprise us so that now surprises are the rule." His team does provide, however, a composite picture of "expert survivors," meaning those past their hundredth birthday, living independently or semi-independently, active in their community, and in relatively good physical and mental health. In the University of Georgia study, this would be a female with a grade-school education who "lives by herself or with her children, has an annual income of $4,000 to $7,000; has vision and hearing problems; takes two medications a day; wants to avoid being institutionalized; is feisty and wants to have her way; and is generally satisfied with life."

The conclusion I draw from looking over the data from these centers is that centenarians exist in all sorts of places—urban and rural, mountainous and flat, coastal and interior, industrialized and nonindustrialized. This finding argues against the possibility that some particular combination of environmental factors—or protection from them—favors longevity and healthful aging. Nor is there any evidence from the population studies that particular foods, supplements, or other substances have anything to do with living to extreme old age. No Shangri-Las or *tangatze* berries stand out in the data.

But before I leave this subject I would like to take you on a quick trip to one of the places I have visited that boasts an unusually high number of centenarians and healthy old people, where birth records are authenticated and scientific research has identified some interesting lifestyle correlations. It is Okinawa, at the southernmost tip of the Japanese islands, itself a subtropical chain of islands that stretches a thousand kilometers across the East China Sea, almost to Taiwan. This archipelago was long an independent, active, and peaceful nation known as the Kingdom of the

Ryukyus, which maintained strong cultural ties to Southeast Asia. Japan annexed the kingdom in 1879 and imposed its culture and language on it, but even today many Okinawans do not consider themselves Japanese. Their physical appearance, diet, and traditions connect them as much to Southeast Asia as to Japan.

Japanese currently enjoy the greatest average life expectancy of any population group on the planet: 79.9 years. And within the Japanese population, Okinawans are the longest-lived subgroup, with an average life expectancy of 81.2 years. I have made three trips to Okinawa in order to investigate some of the factors contributing to their extraordinary longevity and to the numbers of healthy, active old people on the islands.

Okinawa is beautiful, a tropical Pacific paradise, with white sand beaches, turquoise seas, and smog-free skies. Its people are genetically different from Japanese; to me, some of them look Cambodian. They eat a diet quite different from the traditional Japanese diet, with much less salt, more pork, and more tofu, for example. (Pork in Okinawa is simmered a long time to render most of the fat out of it. The tofu has more fat than the usual Japanese versions and is the best I've tasted anywhere.) Okinawans also eat a great many unusual foods and condiments that they believe contribute to health and longevity. Some of them are *mozuku,* a fine, brown seaweed *(Nemacystus decipiens* and *Cladosiphon okamuranus),* usually eaten pickled; *goya,* or bitter melon *(Momordica charantia); ukon,* or turmeric *(Curcuma longa),* commonly drunk as a cold, unsweetened tea; and bright purple—yes, purple—sweet potatoes *(beni imo),* full of antioxidant pigments. Okinawans like alcohol—not the rice wine (sake) of Japan but a local firewater, *awamori,* distilled from rice and aged in ceramic jars. And they drink a lot of tea, usually jasmine tea rather than the green tea of Japan.

Some of my best memories of Okinawa are of exploring the central market in Naha, the capital city, a seemingly endless maze of stands selling the most diverse, colorful, and strange foods, everything from dried poisonous sea snakes to all kinds of edible greens and seaweeds to a profusion of products made from the purple sweet potatoes. This is the ultimate varied diet.

It is tempting to zero in on some of these exotic foods, condiments, and beverages as causes of Okinawan longevity. Bitter melon is worth special attention because it is so much a part of the culture. This strange-looking fruit, something like a warty cucumber, is an effective natural hypoglycemic agent; that is, it lowers blood sugar and may help prevent diabetes and the development of insulin resistance in response to eating quickly digested carbohydrate foods. It is so loved by Okinawans that they not only consume it very frequently in stir-fries but even drink jiggers of the freshly squeezed and distinctly bitter juice. (A chaser of fresh-squeezed sugarcane juice helps it go down easily.) They also make effigies of the fruit to decorate storefronts. I bought a bitter-melon key-chain ornament at a convenience store on the outskirts of Naha, and I've watched the antics of Goya Man on Okinawan television, a popular cartoon character whose body is a bitter melon.

Turmeric is now one of the most intensively studied herbs, attracting a great deal of attention for its anti-inflammatory and cancer-protective effects. Purple pigments in fruits and vegetables boost the body's defenses against oxidative stress and its contribution to aging. (I will explain oxidative stress when I discuss the free-radical theory of aging later in this book. It is the total burden placed on organisms by the oxidation reactions of normal metabolism combined with toxicity from the environment.) I am sure these dietary peculiarities are beneficial to Okinawans, but I doubt they are wholly or even predominantly responsible for their longevity.

Like most traditional people who farm and fish, Okinawans are more physically active than most Western city dwellers. Until recently, obesity was uncommon among them, as were hypertension and atherosclerosis. Okinawans can still breathe clean air and drink clean water, increasingly rare in today's world. They also enjoy another rarity: the cohesiveness of a culture that values community ties and works to include the oldest members in its social fabric.

In fact, Okinawan centenarians and their immediate juniors are regarded as living treasures in this culture, and efforts are made to include them in all community activities. They are regularly to be seen at scientific conferences on aging and longevity, at other civic events, and at locations frequented by Japanese tourists. (Okinawa is an increasingly popular tourist destination for Japanese, especially as it has become known among them as a real-life Shangri-La.) For example, Ogimi Village in the northern part of the main island is known for its centenarians and healthy, active oldsters and advertises itself as a longevity center. I had a memorable lunch there at a restaurant that serves traditional Okinawan health foods, including fresh goya juice. Several women in their late nineties sat around the place, gossiping and laughing, more than willing to share their secrets of healthy living with diners. And across the way, a ninety-five-year-old woman worked in her garden, loosening the earth with a hoe.

"In Okinawa there are none of the age-guessing games that inevitably proved to be the downfall of other Shangri-

La contenders. Every city, town, and village has a family register system *(koseki)* that has been recording reliable birth, marriage, and death statistics since 1879." So write three doctors, two American and one Okinawan, in *The Okinawa Program,* the best book on the subject; all were coinvestigators in the Okinawa Centenarian Study.

Nor are Okinawans reticent about disclosing their ages, a contrast to our culture. In May of 2003 I took my mother, then ninety-two and quite reluctant to have people know that, to Okinawa with me. At a reception for the conference on psychosomatic medicine at which I spoke, a number of the living treasures were present to entertain, as is customary. Each of them, on being introduced to my mother, began the conversation by stating his or her age and asking hers. "Hello, I'm ninety-six; how old are you?" This was quite a cultural shock for my mother, but after a while I think it was refreshing for her to sense the benefits of living in a culture where old age is cause for downright pride.

At the end of the conference, we flew from Naha to an outer island, Ishigaki, even farther removed from noxious influences, and from there we took a boat, with Japanese and Okinawan friends, to Taketomi Island, a tiny place popular with tourists because it is maintained in strictly traditional style: old-fashioned dwellings, no cars, transportation by foot or carts drawn by water buffalo, and plenty of the healthy old people for which Okinawa is now famous. Our little party went to the house of a man who had just celebrated his 101st birthday. He lived alone and appeared to be in good health, except that he was quite deaf. I would have guessed his age at somewhere in the mideighties. A neighbor woman who was in her eighties joined us; she appeared to be about seventy. She took care of the centenarian, making sure he ate properly, for example, and answering the telephone for him; it seemed clear that her devotion to him was a major reason for her own vitality. We all sat on the front step to get to know one another.

On the wall of the old man's house were posted newspaper articles and documents about his *kajimaya* celebration, a unique Okinawan institution.

> [Kajimaya] . . . is arranged by the community to formally mark the transition of one of its citizens to the age of ninety-seven. There is a folk belief in Okinawa that a long-lived person has attained some kind of supernatural power through his or her health and longevity and that others can share in this power by participating in the ceremony. This is called *ayakaru* and it means to share in a person's good luck. People try to touch or shake hands with the long-lived celebrant.

The symbol associated with *kajimaya* is the pinwheel, the child's toy made of folded paper wings pinned to a stick to spin in a breeze. Everyone in attendance carries one. The reason is that Okinawans believe that at ninety-seven one enters one's second childhood, a time to be free of all responsibilities, a time to enjoy life and be taken care of. I learned that a common cause of sibling rivalry in traditional Okinawan households is contention over who will get to take care of the aging parents—not a common problem in the West.

Our centenarian on Taketomi Island certainly seemed to be enjoying himself. If I had to use one word to describe him, it would be "jolly." He beamed, flirted with my mom, saying he wanted an American girlfriend, showed off his citations for being a centenarian, and even pulled out a little stringed instrument to accompany himself while he sang us a song. When my mother asked him his recommendations for long life and health, he replied, "Be happy." He said he loved his island, his home, his friends, and his neighbors, had no regrets, and wanted for nothing.

This is all well and good, but I must mention that Okinawans older than sixty have lived through periods of incredible hardship and social disruption, starting with the years leading up to the Second World War, when the Japanese military occupied and fortified the main island and conscripted its citizens. The Battle of Okinawa, fought from April to June of 1945, was one of the bloodiest engagements of the whole war, the only one fought on Japanese home territory. More people died in it than all those killed in the atomic bombings of Hiroshima and Nagasaki, including 100,000 Okinawan civilians in addition to 107,000 Japanese and Okinawan conscripts. This disaster was followed by the American occupation, which did not end until the territory reverted to Japanese administration in 1972. Since then American military bases have continued to occupy much of Okinawa, a social and political flash point for the islanders.

So, unlike the Shangri-La of *Lost Horizon*, Okinawa has hardly been insulated from the evils of the world, and whatever accounts for the longevity of its citizens must override the stress and social havoc they experienced throughout the second half of the twentieth century. I have been there, I have met the researchers who study the question, and I have read the relevant scientific articles. I think the explanation for the extraordinary phenomenon of healthy aging on these special islands is complex—a combination of genetics, environment, diet, culture, and more, and impossible to disentangle. Nonetheless, I will draw on my experiences in Okinawa in making recommendations for healthy aging later in this book. And, sadly, I must report that Okinawan longevity is now beginning to diminish, as more of its people move to Naha and other population centers, eat Western food, including fast food, and begin to live like the rest of us. In fact, while Okinawan women retain the number one position for longevity in Japan, Okinawan men have fallen to twenty-sixth place in a remarkably short time.

I want to mention briefly another island with a note-worthy population of very old and healthy old people: Sardinia, in the Mediterranean Sea, off the west coast of Italy. You will not find the long-lived Sardinians along the Costa Smeralda or other recently developed beach resorts that cater to tourists and visiting yachts. They live in the remote, mountainous interior and are much less studied and known than their counterparts in Okinawa. A peculiarity of Sardinian longevity is that men and women are represented equally. In all other groups of centenarians that have been studied, women outnumber men by a wide disproportion. It is unknown why Sardinians do not fit this pattern. The healthy aged of Sardinia eat—no surprise—a Mediterranean diet, get plenty of physical activity, breathe clean air, have strong communal ties, and, as in Okinawa, probably do not owe their success to any single factor.

Fountain-of-youth legends are very much alive and well today. At all times and in all cultures people have imagined and searched for substances that could postpone or reverse aging and postpone or negate death. Nectar drunk by both the Hindu and Olympian gods is one example; the word comes from Indo-European roots meaning "beyond death." Human growth hormone (HGH) is one of many substances that people use today in hopes of achieving the same goal.

So pervasive and deep-rooted is the belief in age-reversing substances that an incalculable amount of time, energy, and money has gone and still goes into the discovery, promotion, and marketing of likely candidates. Indeed, their use is a central aspect of contemporary antiaging medicine, which I will discuss in the next chapter.

If you had asked me a few years ago if there were such a thing as a botanical, chemical, or pharmacological fountain of youth, I would have answered with an unequivocal "No!" I might have pointed to the many plants extolled as longevity tonics, especially in Asia, as examples that don't really work as advertised. I have written elsewhere about ginseng, probably the most commercially important of this group. Here I would like to take a critical look at two others that readers may be less familiar with, one a mushroom, the other the root of a plant native to the arctic regions of Eurasia.

Reishi is the Japanese name for *Ganoderma lucidum,* a distinctive, woody mushroom that Chinese call *ling zhi.* In both China and Japan, reishi has a long history of use as a folk medicine and an equally long and rich history as an object of reverence by Taoists, storytellers, and artists. Many colorful names exist for it in both cultures and in Korea, among them, Mushroom of Immortality, Tree of Life Mushroom, and Ten-Thousand-Year Mushroom, all suggesting life-extending properties. Many centuries-old Chinese paintings depict reishi; the mushroom is immediately recognizable by its unique cap (usually heart shaped, with concentric zones, and so shiny that it appears to be coated with lacquer). In these paintings, sages and immortals often hold the mushroom in their hands. Images of it are carved on doors of the Imperial Palace in Beijing, embroidered on robes once worn by Chinese emperors, woven into fine silk tapestries, and painted on valuable scrolls that adorned palace walls.

Ganoderma lucidum is a member of the polypore family of mushrooms, the shelf or bracket fungi that grow on living and dead trees and help recycle organic matter in forests. Reishi is certainly beautiful and attractive, coming as it does in a great variety of colors and forms; moreover, it does not rot. Perhaps that characteristic led Taoist shamans, obsessed with finding longevity herbs and secrets of immortality, to take up its use. Reishi is nontoxic, but it is too woody and too bitter to be eaten as food. It can be chopped and boiled into a medicinal tea, and, based on observation of its effects in this form, Chinese medical philosophers classified it as a superior drug and recommended it for increasing resistance and extending life. Once rare in the wild, which may have enhanced its reputation, it is easily cultivated and now in large-scale production in China, Korea, Japan, and North America.

The medical literature contains numerous research reports on reishi, including results of both animal and human studies. Based on that work, some Western doctors now recommend it as having significant anti-inflammatory effects without any of the side effects of anti-inflammatory drugs. It also enhances immune function, making it a useful adjunctive therapy for people with cancer and AIDS. Consumer demand has created a brisk market for reishi and products made from it. You will find them in every health-food store.

Unfortunately, none of the research on reishi documents any life-extending properties. Taking a natural anti-inflammatory agent might be useful, because many age-related diseases seem to be rooted in inappropriate and persistent inflammation (see Chapter 9). Enhancing immunity is also a good idea, given so many environmental assaults on health. But I must conclude that there is no scientific basis for the ancient Chinese belief that *Ganoderma lucidum* is a fungal fountain of youth.

Another plant candidate to possess wondrous powers is

arctic root, also known as golden root and rose root, the underground part of *Rhodiola rosea,* native to high latitudes of the Northern Hemisphere. A relative of the sedums and the jade plant, it is a perennial with a thick root that is fragrant when freshly cut. In Scandinavia, Siberia, Mongolia, and China, among other places, traditional peoples prized the root as a remedy to enhance physical strength and endurance, treat chronic diseases, enhance fertility, and ensure the birth of healthy children. Bouquets of the roots are still presented to couples as wedding presents in remote Siberian villages.

In modern times, Russian scientists confirmed the botanical identity of the source of golden root, studied its chemistry, and investigated its properties in both animals and humans. More recent research is ongoing in Sweden. *Rhodiola rosea* root contains a group of distinctive compounds called rosavins that are at least partially responsible for the plant's remarkable properties. These include antifatigue, antistress, anticancer, antioxidant, immune-enhancing, and sexually stimulating effects. In addition, arctic root enhances the activity of a number of neurotransmitters in the brain, which may explain its reputation for promoting mental clarity and cognition. It may also improve mood and memory and reduce the risk of age-related memory loss. Its toxicity is low.

I feel comfortable predicting that arctic root will become better known in Europe and America, that scientific research will continue to document its benefits, and that it may prove to counteract some of the losses of central nervous system functioning that occur with age. I have taken it myself and like its effects. But it is hardly a reverser of aging.

Arctic root, reishi, ginseng, and many other natural products are known as tonics or adaptogens, the latter term coined by two Soviet pharmacologists in 1968 to describe nontoxic substances that nonspecifically increase the resistance of an organism to a wide range of harmful influences and normalize its functions. Practitioners of traditional Chinese medicine would say that tonics strengthen the defensive sphere of function of the body. Western pharmacologists would look to modulation of immunity as the mechanism of action. Effective tonics have a secure place in a healthy lifestyle, one designed to reduce risks of chronic disease and increase the chances of a healthy, productive old age. I recommend learning about them, experimenting with them, and finding one or several to take every day as a long-term strategy. And even while I make this recommendation and faithfully take my arctic root, reishi, and other Asian tonic mushrooms, I know that none of these substances will reverse, halt, or slow the aging process itself. The repertory of herbal tonics and adaptogens, extensive as it is, does not contain the long-sought fountain of youth.

So let's turn our attention to stronger stuff, specifically to hormones, those powerful compounds produced in the body that regulate basic life processes of metabolism, growth, and maturation. Many hormones are used in medicine, and many are touted as antiaging agents. Might the fountain that we are searching for be spewing hormone supplements?

The best candidate in this group is human growth hormone (HGH), known to science since the 1920s, when it was discovered in the pituitary gland. Disorders of growth hormone production were recognized long before the hormone itself: giantism and acromegaly from too much and dwarfism from too little. (Giantism occurs with excessive HGH production in childhood; acromegaly, marked by enlargement of the head, hands, and feet, occurs when too much of the hormone is present in adults.) When human growth hormone became available as an extract of cadaver pituitary glands, effective treatment of dwarfism became possible. But this form of treatment came to a crashing halt in the early 1980s when some patients developed Creutzfeldt-Jakob disease (CJD), the human variant of spongiform encephalopathy that is equivalent to mad cow disease in cows. CJD is caused by infectious protein particles (prions). Cadaver pituitaries are attached to remnants of hypothalamus, the part of the brain that produces compounds that control secretion of pituitary hormones. Some of that brain tissue came from people infected with CJD, and CJD prions wound up in the growth hormone preparations given to patients with dwarfism.

Fortunately, in 1985, after a brief hiatus, a noncadaver source of HGH became available, manufactured with recombinant DNA technology. In fact, it became widely available, marketed by both genetic engineering and pharmaceutical companies. This encouraged physicians to look for other applications of HGH, even though the hormone has to be given by daily injection over long periods of time and is very expensive. The yearly cost of treatment is about $14,000, and the companies producing it are not in competition, so the cost stays high.

The first new use of the manufactured form of HGH was the treatment of short children. This immediately raised concerns that a powerful hormone was being used for cosmetic rather than medical purposes. Some short children may be deficient in HGH; most are producing all they need and are simply genetically short. If you give them daily injections of HGH up to the time their long bones mature, they will gain height. The treatment appears safe but remains controversial.

Much more controversial is the more recent assertion that growth hormone can reverse age-associated changes in body composition and therefore act as a general rejuvenator. Claims for these properties of HGH are all over the Internet and in many books and articles aimed at both health professionals and the public. All of them trace back to the publication on June 5, 1990, of an article by Dr. Daniel Rudman et al. in the *New England Journal of Medicine*. The title of that article was "Effects of Human Growth Hormone in Men over 60 Years Old." Dr. Rudman, then a researcher at the Medical College of Wisconsin, studied twenty-one healthy men, aged sixty-one to eighty-one. He gave twelve of them thrice-weekly injections of HGH for six months and observed a significant increase in lean body mass and bone density and a decrease in adipose (fatty) tissue mass compared to the untreated controls.

Scientists have long known that production of growth hormone in the pituitary declines with aging. That in turn causes decreased production of another hormone, IGF-1 (insulin-like growth factor), that regulates metabolism and is needed for normal growth. (The liver produces IGF-1 in response to stimulation by growth hormone.) Rudman's hypothesis was that "declining activity of the growth hormone–insulin-like growth factor 1 (IGF-1) axis with advancing age may contribute to the decrease in lean body mass and the increase in mass of adipose tissue that occur with aging." Results of his study were consistent with the hypothesis. In the treated men, IGF-1 levels rose into the youthful range, lean body mass increased by 8.8 percent, adipose-tissue mass decreased by 14.4 percent, and the density of bone in the lumbar spine increased by 1.6 percent.

What is the significance of those results? Loss of muscle and gain of fat are certainly two of the most visible changes that occur in the aged. They account for the sunken faces, thin limbs, and potbellies of many older people and are probably more distressing to them than more serious but less visible changes in internal organs. Furthermore, loss of lean body mass may initiate a vicious cycle of change in body composition, because skeletal muscles constitute a metabolic furnace that burns calories much more efficiently than adipose tissue. Anyone wanting to lose or control weight should, in addition to eating less and exercising more, try to increase lean body mass—by weight training, for example—in order to keep the metabolic furnace burning bright. The more muscle mass you lose and the more fat you put on, the more fat you will put on. All of this is controlled by the growth hormone–IGF-1 axis of hormonal activity. The decline of growth hormone secretion in the elderly has been termed the "somatopause"—analogous to menopause in women—with hormone replacement suggested as the remedy in both cases.

It seems incredible that one article reporting a short-term study in such a small population could have launched an entire antiaging movement based on the administration of human growth hormone, but such is the case. If you enter "HGH" in your favorite Internet search engine, you will be overwhelmed by the number of sites promoting and selling growth hormone and related products; most of them cite the 1990 Rudman study as the scientific basis for their claims.

Here are some statements that I've collected from these sites:

- Basically, anything that goes on in your body is in some way tied to HGH. This is why HGH is often called the "fountain of youth." Elevated HGH levels are what make you feel young again.
- Research into HGH shows that aging may be preventable to a certain extent . . . our body is very capable at the age

of forty to have the same makeup as we did at the age of twenty.

- While numerous studies have been done on the effects of HGH injections, the most groundbreaking study was done by Dr. Daniel Rudman and published in *The New England Journal of Medicine.*

- HGH is truly an amazing substance that has been shown to have numerous clinically proven benefits. In fact, studies published in *The New England Journal of Medicine* prove that HGH can shed body fat, increase muscle tone, boost your energy, reduce wrinkles, help you sleep better, improve sex drive and performance, improve immune and heart function, improve brain function.

- Research has shown that virtually every adult is HGH deficient. By the age of forty you already have "elderly" levels of HGH production, down as much as 50 percent of youthful levels. The earlier you address declining HGH levels the better.

    And it's never too late. Dr. Daniel Rudman, M.D., of the Medical College of Wisconsin, conducted a groundbreaking HGH research study in 1990. . . .

- Restore your looks, health, energy, and physical abilities to the levels of a robust young adult! Men and women: become immune to the passage of time . . . replenish your body's lost levels of HGH!

If you visit these sites, you will note that many of them are, in fact, selling not HGH but a variety of pills, powders, oral sprays, and homeopathic remedies supposed to promote the release of HGH from the pituitary. All of them are bogus. Growth hormone releasers do exist and may be a better therapeutic option than HGH itself, but they are not to be found on the Internet. I will tell you about them shortly.

I also found companies selling actual HGH in injectable form and at the expected price, often combined in even more expensive antiaging hormone cocktails with testosterone and human chorionic gonadotropin (HCG), a substance produced by the placenta in pregnancy and obtained from the urine of pregnant women, also supposed to maintain youthfulness.

It is hard to obtain unbiased information on the benefits, dangers, and appropriate uses of HGH because most of the doctors and other experts who talk and write about it are in one way or another involved with its distribution and marketing. For an objective view from an unbiased expert, I turned to Seymour (Si) Reichlin, an eminent neuroendocrinologist and researcher who happens to be my neighbor. Before he moved to the Arizona desert, Si, now eighty, was chief of the Division of Endocrinology at Tufts–New England Medical Center, where he studied control of the pituitary gland by the brain and where he gained renown as one of our foremost experts on that gland. He has no financial interest in promoting any anti-aging product.

"The pituitary secretes HGH episodically, every ninety minutes, more at night than during the day," Si says. "The magnitude of these spikes peaks in the late teens and declines with age. Giving an injection of HGH once a day is convenient, but it is very different from the natural cycle of secretion.

"Larger studies of HGH treatment continue to show that it increases muscle mass and decreases body fat, but up to one-third of subjects have significant side effects, like joint pain and carpal tunnel syndrome. [Growth hormone increases the thickness of connective tissue throughout the body.] There have been some cases of hypertension and rarer cases of cerebral edema [brain swelling]. So there is a definite downside to HGH treatment. And there is a theoretical concern about increased risk of cancer, because we see more cancer in people with acromegaly. Finally, there is a change in glucose tolerance, with a push toward the development of diabetes.

"So what we have now is a potent substance with potentially serious side effects being used promiscuously. Maybe there is a germ of something good in the current pattern of HGH treatment, but it may only be helpful if you take it for a very long time, at great expense, and any effects wear off as soon as you stop using it."

I asked Si if he would take it himself. "No," he replied without hesitation, "only as part of a clinical trial, not otherwise. You have to be careful not to give too much, and you have to monitor the response."

Si Reichlin is most skeptical about claims that supplemental HGH can extend life. "That's highly unlikely," he says. "It may reverse the metabolic accompaniments of aging, but work in mice suggests that it may actually shorten life, so you'll look better but die sooner." He also points out that exercise can produce the same favorable changes in body composition as growth hormone. "No one tells you that," he says.

I also talked with Si about growth hormone releasers, an interesting area of research. The hypothalamus makes a well-known growth hormone–releasing factor (GHRF) that controls the cycle of pituitary secretion of HGH, but other releasing factors are known, one a hormone called ghrelin secreted by the stomach that helps regulate appetite. Orally active analogs of growth hormone–releasing factors are known. One pill a day may restore the normal cyclic production of HGH that occurs in youth. "That I would consider taking," Si said, "but I have my doubts that it will become available. The pharmaceutical companies that hold patents on these orally active growth hormone releasers also make HGH and are getting their $14,000 a year and more from each patient taking it. Why should they undercut their sales?"

Human growth hormone is probably the best approximation of a fountain of youth now available. Certainly, many claims to that effect are being made for it. But, as Si Reichlin warns, "You're not going to get the truth about it from people making money off it. I wish the community of antiaging doctors would carry out proper dose-response studies and careful analysis of benefits and complications, but they are already convinced that HGH is effective and free of complications. There is now strong motivation *not* to do these kinds of studies. In my view, the status of HGH therapy can be regarded as similar to that of estrogen replacement therapy in postmenopausal women: there may be some benefits, but there may also be an undesirable downside."

Telomerase and stem cells suggest theoretical possibilities for antiaging treatments of the future, but doctors can't prescribe them and you won't find them for sale on the Internet. That brings us to the subject of the next chapter, the rise of a new field of medicine devoted to the reversal of aging.

3

ANTIAGING MEDICINE

Aging Is a Process. So Is Reversing It

—Sign on a bus stop in midtown Manhattan
advertising a dermatology clinic specializing
in Botox injections (2004)

Antiaging medicine is nothing new. What is remarkable today is its growth into an organized field, with journals, annual meetings, and a concerted attempt by leaders to have it recognized as a legitimate specialty of orthodox medicine.

In the past, individual doctors have promoted various rejuvenation techniques, many of them derived from ideas and practices going back to antiquity. It is useful to look at the prescriptions of today's antiaging doctors in historical context. For example, the contemporary infatuation with hormones and antioxidants is squarely in the tradition of using magical substances, including mushrooms of immortality, developed over thousands of years in the Taoist traditions of China and Korea. Caloric restriction, a proven method of extending life and enhancing health in many animal species, harks back to the austerities practiced by sadhus in India from ancient times in order to achieve maximum life and vitality.

One prominent theme in the historical record is that aging occurs because of the loss over time of some vital principle or essence. The Taoists equated this with emissions of semen in men and taught secret techniques to initiates intended to allow sexual orgasm without ejaculation and thereby increase longevity. Other philosophers talked about the gradual drying up of inner moisture and recommended consuming substances like pearl and coral to replenish it. Some identified breath with the vital principle and urged people to gain control of it and slow it down in order to live longer. Roger Bacon, the thirteenth-century English scientist, thought the breath of young virgins could replenish the vital essence of old men and recommended spending time in their company. "Curiously, breathing the air of young virgin boys was never mentioned as an antiaging therapy for older women."

A contemporary spin on this theme is the suggestion that laziness is the key to longevity, because it conserves life energy. In their recent book, *The Joy of Laziness,* a German father-and-daughter team of health experts argue that avoiding exercise and stress and limiting ambition can extend life by slowing down the rate at which you consume the finite amount of vital energy you were born with. One reviewer comments: "What a practical book! It takes away your bad conscience when you're unable to get up on a Saturday morning!"

In the twentieth century, with the development of and public enthusiasm for medical technology, rejuvenation techniques evolved into scientific therapies or at least into therapies appearing to be scientific. One of the earliest, most famous, and most persistent is "cellular therapy" or "live cell therapy," once available only to the very rich at a private clinic in Switzerland, now offered in Mexico and other countries (not in the United States) at somewhat less expense. Its major proponent was a Swiss surgeon, Paul Niehans (1882–1971), whose technique was to harvest cells from the organs of fetal sheep and inject them into the buttocks of clients. His theory was that cells from organs of an unborn animal, high in vitality, would somehow get to the corresponding organs of an adult human and somehow rejuvenate them.

Niehans practiced at the Clinique La Prairie in Clarens-Montreux, which attracted many famous clients from the 1930s on, among them Winston Churchill, Konrad Adenauer, Dwight Eisenhower, Somerset Maugham, and other political leaders, artists, and movie stars. Charlie Chaplin made many visits to the Clinique and attributed his fathering two children in his seventies to Niehans's treatment. Pope Pius XII took the injections near the end of his life in 1953 and was so pleased with the results that he admitted Niehans to membership in the Papal Academy of Sciences. The Clinique La Prairie (CLP) is still in operation, offering weeklong "revitalization packages" that include medical tests, spa services, and two injections of what are now called "CLP extracts." The weekly cost, depending on class of room, ranges from $27,000 to $34,000.

Over the years, cellular therapy has evolved. The CLP extracts used today at the Clinique La Prairie are no longer suspensions of actual cells but freeze-dried extracts of cells, mainly from fetal sheep livers, guaranteed to be free of viruses, low in allergenic potential, and high in mysterious "senescent cell activating factors (SCAF)." These are conceived as "embryonic substance(s) [that] restore the responsiveness of senescent cells to growth factors by restoring growth factor receptors; by such treatment the cells acquire the morphology and physiology of 'younger' cells." Is this science, or is it a modern way of packaging and injecting the revitalizing breath of young virgins?

Since Dr. Niehans's death, the Clinique La Prairie has affiliated with several orthodox medical institutions in Germany and cites research done at those centers that purports to prove injected fetal cells and cell extracts do, in fact, reach their intended target organs rather than being destroyed by the recipient's immune system. Proponents now claim that the injections not only stimulate general rejuvenation but also treat specific diseases, including cancer, AIDS, Down syndrome, obesity, amyotrophic lateral sclerosis (ALS), and Alzheimer's disease. Needless to say, the mainstream medical community rejects these claims, if it even pays attention to them at all. The Web site of a "holistic life extension center" in Mexico says:

> It is important to note that those who practice "orthodox" medicine will be quite vocal in their opposition to this "unorthodox" treatment. Here's the reason: The greatest enemies of Live-Cell Treatment are the large and powerful pharmaceutical companies whose sole existence rel[ies] on pill manufacturing. If we are able to cure a condition, then suddenly big business is in trouble, with its very existence threatened. Live-Cell Therapy is not a drug-based treatment.

Here is the crux of the immense difference between practitioners of antiaging medicine and their more conventional colleagues: The former are using methods and making claims that the latter consider unsupported by scientific evidence. Most of those methods may be relatively harmless except to the bank accounts of clients; some may not be. (I have not seen any negative effects from the use of live cell therapy.) Proponents also portray themselves as under attack by conventional medicine, which is out to suppress them as intellectual and economic threats.

With the founding in 1993 of the American Academy of Anti-Aging Medicine—A4M for short—practitioners of antiaging medicine found a home and a power base. A4M claims 12,500 physician members from seventy-three countries. It publishes textbooks, journals, and magazines, lobbies for recognition of itself by the American Medical Association, and holds huge conferences, both in the United States and around the world (Spain, Singapore, Mexico). It also produces books for consumers with titles like *New Anti-Aging Secrets for Maximum Lifespan, Hormones of Youth, Grow Young with HGH,* and *Stopping the Clock.*

A4M is the brainchild of two physicians, Robert Goldman and Ronald Klatz. Goldman is a former competitive gymnast, bodybuilder, martial artist, and sports medicine doctor who did research early in his career on anabolic steroids. Klatz, also a sports medicine doctor, did research on brain resuscitation and is the inventor of a number of medical devices. The major academic affiliation of both has been the Central America Health Sciences University in Belize. Neither man is formally trained in geriatrics or is part of the society of biogerontologists, the scientific experts on aging.

In fact, there is a definite schism between biogerontologists and A4M, more visible since the publication in 2002 of the "Position Statement on Human Aging" by leading biogerontologists. Here is a representative quote from that article:

There has been a resurgence and proliferation of health care providers and entrepreneurs who are promoting antiaging products and lifestyle changes that they claim will slow, stop, or reverse the processes of aging. Even though in most cases there is little or no scientific basis for these claims, the public is spending vast sums of money on these products and lifestyle changes, some of which may be harmful.

To counter these charges, Dr. Klatz sent an "Urgent Message" to all members of A4M. It began:

The American Academy of Anti-Aging Medicine writes you today on a matter of urgent importance. *Anti-aging medicine is under an unwarranted and unprecipitated attack.* **A premeditated, malicious, and deliberate disinformation campaign directed at dismantling the single most unified group of innovative physicians and scientists in America is now underway.** A powerful old-boy network is investing enormous time, personnel, and financial resources on destroying today's most successful, most popular, and fastest-growing medical society.

To get a sense of this division in medical and scientific thinking and practice, I went to Las Vegas in December of 2003 to attend the Eleventh Annual Anti-Aging Conference and Exposition, which filled the Venetian Resort and an adjoining exhibit hall. After a brief greeting to the audience of about 2,500 physicians, Ron Klatz introduced a representative of Primedia, the company that has produced and managed the A4M's conferences. He was not expecting her to say what she did.

She announced that her company would be parting ways

with A4M after this event and, in fact, would be putting on a "next generation" of "science-based" longevity medicine conferences in the fall of 2004. She explained that these new conferences would have a peer-review program committee "to ensure that all presentations are ethical, educational, and evidence based." Then she introduced an unscheduled speaker, Dr. L. Stephen Coles from the University of California, Los Angeles, head of the Los Angeles Gerontology Research Group and chairman of that very program committee. Dr. Coles gave a brief and provocative talk, one most unwelcome to many in the crowd.

He began by showing slides of the title pages of the "Position Statement on Human Aging" and related articles and told the audience of antiaging doctors that there were no such things as antiaging medicines at present, although scientists were working to develop them. He invited people to attend the upcoming, more scientific conferences, then left the podium quickly.

The effect on the audience of this bombshell was unsettling. The 2,500 doctors in attendance had just been told they were on a wrong path and wasting their time, energy, and money.

Drs. Goldman and Klatz were clearly blindsided by Coles's appearance and hostile remarks. Klatz rallied his audience by telling them, "We attract the best clinicians in the world."

"I couldn't disagree more with the first speaker," he went on. "We know that antiaging therapeutics are very helpful and powerful. I find it repugnant that fifty-one scientists signed a statement saying there is no such thing as antiaging medicine, especially when most of them are on the dole from the National Institute of Aging. This controversy is not scientific—it represents political competition from the gerontological establishment. The fact is that antiaging medicine is a revenue generator and a great way to practice. It makes money for the doctor. You can quadruple your revenue, especially if you add preventive medical screenings. This market is growing by 9 percent a year." Klatz's implication was that biogerontologists are jealous of this success.

"How many of you use human growth hormone in your practice?" he asked. About half of the people in the room raised their hands. "That's great!" he said.

"And how many of you have seen any adverse reactions from human growth hormone?" No hands went up. "HGH is so effective," Klatz continued, "and research on it is so strong; tens of thousands of docs are using it, and we've yet to see any serious adverse effects. . . .

"If antiaging medicine is not real, why are people living longer, happier, and more healthful lives?" Klatz asked. "We are on the verge of practical immortality, with life spans in excess of a hundred years. Fifty percent of baby boomers can live to a hundred and beyond. Telomerase and stem cells and cloning will take us to a hundred and twenty and beyond. Soon we will be the Ageless Society."

Dr. Klatz received a standing ovation.

There followed an inspirational keynote address by John Gray, author of *Men Are from Mars, Women Are from Venus* (and countless variations on that theme). His talk was titled "Gender-Specific Diet, Nutrition, and Weight-Management to Attain Balanced Brain Chemistry, and Optimal Health." At various points, he got the audience to stand and do vigorous movements and breathing exercises to move energy around their bodies.

Bob Goldman then presented A4M's Infinity Award—its highest honor—posthumously to Dr. Robert Atkins, of Atkins diet fame. His widow accepted the award as Goldman told her that "people are realizing he was right all along." A five-minute video was shown of Dr. Atkins, in which he said, "My diet works 100 percent of the time."

Dr. Goldman then gave his own inspirational speech, announcing that "We can now de-age people." He showed many slides of bodybuilding seniors, and throughout his presentation I noted an emphasis on appearance—on body aesthetics and muscle definition, among other things. "We now see people in their eighties working out, which is great," he said, "and tomorrow's hundred-year-old will be like today's sixty-year-old." He then went through a long list of medical breakthroughs coming soon to your local antiaging medical center: "Stem cells will be one of our magic bullets—we'll be able to program them to regrow tissue where it's needed." Developments in nanotechnology—machines so tiny you will need a microscope to see them—will enable us to restore vision. There will be new drug delivery systems for restorative hormones, therapeutic cloning to produce new organs to replace old ones, gene therapies to extend life, and even bionic interfaces between our brains and computers. The goal is to come out like Arnold Schwarzenegger, a friend of Goldman's and his hero. "He not only has great genetics but also the knowledge and the motivation. . . .

"You are all part of a global paradigm shift," Goldman told his enthusiastic audience. "Attitude is everything."

I found a number of the plenary presentations interesting, especially one on the role of chronic inflammation as a common root of age-related diseases and another on novel treatments for neurodegenerative diseases like Parkinson's, Alzheimer's, and ALS; both emphasized dietary modification as a treatment strategy. Then the session was over, and we were invited to visit the exhibit hall. Dr. Klatz cautioned us to remember that the exhibits were independent of the scientific conference and that A4M should not be judged by the nature of the exhibitors it attracted.

It attracted a lot of them. The hall was full of vendors selling devices, services, and supplements. A distributor of human growth hormone had the largest and most prominent display. Many exhibitors promoted their brands of antioxidants, fish oils, and miracle herbs. Some of what was offered struck me as legitimate, much seemed pseudo-scientific—devices for reading and adjusting energy fields, for example. I was exhausted after walking up and down the aisles and was delighted when I got to a far corner and saw friends of mine from Alaska. They were offering samples of their wild salmon, which is high in desirable omega-3 fatty acids and low in contaminants. They had never been to an A4M event before.

I had dinner with them that night, and they told me about their experience. "It's funny," one of them said. "We're the only people offering real food here, and people don't know what to make of it. They keep trying to figure out what our gimmick is."

There were a great many gimmicks offered for sale in the exhibit hall, including devices to balance the human aura. Most of them would have both amused and appalled my colleagues in conventional medicine.

For two days, I dropped in on lectures, chatted informally with A4M members, talked with Ron Klatz and Bob Goldman about the history and present course of the academy, returned to the exhibits, and tried to avoid the smoke and noise of the Venetian's casino and get decent food—not easy tasks. I also tried to sort out my thoughts about antiaging medicine.

Most of the A4M members I met were sincere practitioners delighted to be involved in an exciting new field. Many seemed to me to have come to that field after becoming fed up with the nature of conventional medicine. Like many doctors in America today, they had tired of the paperwork, rising costs, and diminishing returns of practicing orthopedic surgery or obstetrics or gastroenterology. They had discovered in antiaging medicine a way to attract different kinds of patients who were much easier to work with: the worried well rather than the really sick. Moreover, these patients tend to be educated, affluent, and willing to pay out of pocket for tests, products, and services not covered by insurance. And, as Dr. Klatz pointed out in his opening address, there is good money to be made on the tests, products, and services. These were clinicians, not researchers; practitioners, not scientists.

In much of what I heard at the conference, I noted a failure to distinguish age-related diseases from the aging process itself. It is one thing to work toward the prevention, early diagnosis, reversal, and modification of diseases that become more likely as people age. It is something else entirely to talk about preventing or reversing the process of aging. When the biogerontologists say there is no such thing as antiaging medicine, they mean that there is no way to stop the clock or reverse the aging process. They do not mean that doctors should not do everything they can to help people live longer, more active, and more comfortable lives by minimizing the ravages of age-related diseases. In fact, the latter approach, known as "compression of morbidity," is quite respectable scientifically; the central idea is to delay the onset of age-related disease and inevitable decline without worrying about extending life. The amount of time people would have to spend sick and suffering a poor quality of life would thus be compressed, giving them more years of active life and sparing society the costs of maintaining so many chronically ill old people.

I must agree with Dr. Coles that at present there are no effective antiaging medicines. Scientific evidence is incomplete at best, and totally lacking at worst, for all of the products and services I heard about in the lectures and saw on display in the exhibit hall. Most of those products and services are costly; some may be harmful.

Finally, I am dismayed by the emphasis on appearance in antiaging medicine. This is apparent not just in the use of senior bodybuilders as models of healthy aging but in the prominent inclusion of cosmetic surgery in the American Academy of Anti-Aging Medicine and its conferences and publications. Presentations at an A4M conference in June of 2003 included one titled "Plastic Surgery and Anti-Aging: A Natural Combination." At the Las Vegas event, there was one on "Office Based Non-Surgical Cosmetic Therapies for the Anti-Aging Physician: Botox, Facial Fillers, Laser, Cosmeceuticals" and another on "Factors Associated with Efficacy and Satisfaction of Superficial Chemical Peel in Asian Skin." To my mind, all this represents attempts to deny or mask the outward signs of aging. It is nonacceptance of aging—one of the great obstacles to growing old gracefully, as I said earlier.

If you are tempted by the promises of antiaging medicine, whether from practitioners, clinics, or salespersons, I would advise you to use it selectively. Always assess the potential for harm of any intervention offered to you. Then try to evaluate the evidence for any claimed benefits. Weigh potential benefits against possible risks, including exorbitant costs. Get second opinions from doctors who are not part of the antiaging enterprise. If you do go on some treatment regimen, set a time limit for judging whether it does you any good—say, three to six months. Then determine if it was worth the cost.

Before I leave this subject, I want to warn you that the promises you will hear from practitioners of antiaging medicine are going to become more extravagant in coming years. I have described the schism that exists between biogerontologists and the American Academy of Anti-Aging Medicine. There is now another schism that has developed within the ranks of the scientists who study aging that will have an impact on this field. A number of hard-core molecular biologists claim to have identified genetic mechanisms that control the aging process as well as ways of manipulating them. These researchers very much believe that the biological clock *can* be stopped or turned back, and as antiaging doctors learn about this work, they will use it to their advantage.

At a time when genomics is so much on the cutting edge of science, it would seem obvious to look for genes that control aging or confer longevity. The official line of biogerontologists is that such genes cannot exist for the simple reason that natural selection works only until the time that organisms reproduce. It cannot select for or preserve genes that affect life beyond reproduction, except for some minimal time thereafter when parents are needed to ensure the survival of offspring. This is consistent with the fact that nature is very much concerned with perpetuation of life at the species level but cares little for individuals once they have passed on their genes. It is the trade-off I noted earlier between sex and death. By choosing a reproductive strategy that increases the likelihood of the survival of species, nature commits to the death of individuals and does not concern itself with how individuals age. Jay Olshansky has stated this fact most succinctly: "There are no death or aging genes—period." Leonard Hayflick has expressed strong doubt that any dramatic increases in human life span are possible. He has also said, "There are no genes for aging. I'll say that categorically."

I began to hear different views when I attended an International Conference on Longevity held in Okinawa in November of 2001. Thomas Perls, then director of the New England Centenarian Study, told the audience that human bodies are designed to last eighty years or so if their owners avoid the common lifestyle pitfalls that cause premature disability and death (skydiving and smoking, for example). "But," he said, "to live into the nineties and beyond, you probably need genetic booster rockets." He described his search for them by scanning the genomes of pairs of unusually long-lived siblings. Perls and his colleagues identified a region on human chromosome 4 containing several hundred genes that appeared to be the right target area. This work generated a lot of media attention and encouraged Perls to join a biotechnology company to close in on the genes and develop drugs to influence them.

(Some longevity genes may affect the transport of cholesterol in the body. In 2003 researchers reported finding a genetic variation in centenarians and near centenarians that leads to larger-size lipoprotein particles, the carriers of cholesterol. People with this genotype also have higher levels of HDL cholesterol, the good kind that offers protection from heart attacks.)

Michael Rose, an evolutionary biologist at the University of California, Irvine, told how he had tripled the life span of fruit flies by the simple strategy of not allowing them to reproduce until they were older. This encourages selection for the ability to reproduce at older ages, which requires good health at older ages. He has focused on a small number of genes that appear to be involved in this process: genes that affect basic metabolism.

This research dovetails neatly with investigations of caloric restriction as a means of extending life and improving health in animals, and points to an intimate relationship between metabolic rate and reproduction and between reproduction and aging. In cold-blooded animals, life span can be increased by dropping ambient temperature, thereby slowing all body functions, but in warm-blooded species the only proven method of life extension is restriction of caloric intake, an intervention sometimes called "caloric restriction with adequate nutrition."

Experiments going back to the 1930s have shown that feeding laboratory animals about a third fewer calories than they would eat freely, without causing malnutrition, can dramatically increase their longevity. Mice in this situation may live four years longer than normal, a 50 percent increase. Moreover, they remain much healthier than their freely eating counterparts, showing an equally dramatic delay in the onset of age-related diseases. This work has been repeated in rats and many other species, including, most recently, monkeys. Underfed monkeys live longer and have much lower risks of cancer, heart problems, and other maladies. We do not yet have comparable data from humans, but there is every reason to think that experiments in us would give the same results. Already, a number of advocates of caloric restriction have published life-extension diet plans, and many people are following them.

The problem for most of us is that eating and food give too much immediate pleasure and satisfaction to be sacrificed for the distant goal of longer life. Might there be another way of attaining that goal by understanding the mechanism by which caloric restriction affects longevity?

If an organism is to reproduce, it must have adequate

nutritional reserves to produce germ cells, embryos, and young. If those reserves are not available, reproductive systems shut down. (It is well known, for example, that female athletes with a low percentage of body fat stop menstruating.) Caloric restriction is a form of stress for an organism, an indication that the environment might be turning hostile and less favorable for reproduction. In response, certain genes become active in order to slow metabolism and increase body defenses, hedging against a time when conditions will become more favorable. This strategy must have appeared early in the course of evolution, because it is common to many organisms. When food is scarce, all creatures great and small slow down, live longer, and postpone reproduction until times get better.

Scientists are busily studying the genes involved in this response in organisms as diverse as yeasts, worms, and humans, and they are finding broad commonalities across these species. Some of the most provocative work has involved a species of nematode, a tiny worm no wider than a thread and only a millimeter long with the many-millimeters-long name of *Caenorhabditis elegans*. This tiny creature has the distinction of being the first organism to have all its genes sequenced. It has more than 19,000 of them and, remarkably, has 40 percent of them in common with humans.

C. elegans has a normal life span of twenty days. Researchers have been able to triple that by tinkering with various genes, especially ones that control metabolism in the creature's brain. The most dramatic effect follows from changes to a gene called *daf-2* that appears to be a master regulator of many other genes involved with metabolism and defense. Active genes instruct cells to produce particular proteins that orchestrate the functions of life. The *daf-2* protein is a hormone receptor that controls the activities of as many as a hundred other genes. Cynthia Kenyon, a structural biologist at the University of California, San Francisco, has extended the life span of *C. elegans* to 125 days by modifying this master gene. Not only that: her long-lived worms remain robust and healthy until the end. Kenyon has also recently cofounded a company called Elixir Pharmaceuticals that intends to create an antiaging pill.

The reason for her entry into the biotech industry is clear. The hormonal system controlled by *daf-2* in *C. elegans* is the same one that influences longevity in fruit flies and mice and has an exact correspondence in humans. Insulin is a principal player in the human system, along with its cousin IGF-1 (insulin-like growth factor).

When I was in medical school, I learned that insulin regulates levels of blood sugar, allowing glucose to enter cells to be metabolized. Insufficient production of it (type 1 diabetes) or insufficient receptors for it (type 2 diabetes) both cause persistently elevated blood sugar, accelerated development of cardiovascular disease, and a variety of other serious problems. Today, the role of insulin in the human body appears much more complex and interesting. It is a master control of the processing, storage, and distribution of energy. Disturbances in insulin production or the response to it may be at the root of obesity, the degenerative changes that occur in many tissues with aging, and even the development of cancer. Insulin and related hormones may also be key determinants of life span. When asked about the possibility of extending human life span by changing a gene corresponding to *daf-2* in *C. elegans,* Cynthia Kenyon replied:

> We might be able to, we don't know; but it's possible that we could change a human gene and double our life

span. I don't know if that's true, but we can't rule that out. I think that the difference between the life spans of different species may boil down to the activity of master regulator genes, like the *daf-2* receptor. . . . I doubt that humans have special genes for longevity that the worms don't have.

Another line of investigation is the search for substances that mimic the effects of products of the master regulators. In yeasts, the gene that mediates the response to caloric restriction is called *sir-2* (for "silent information regulator"), and it, too, has an exact counterpart in humans. A team at Harvard University screened a large number of chemicals, looking for ones that might activate *sir-2* without semistarvation. They found a promising candidate in resveratrol, a compound that was in the news a few years ago as the component of red wine largely responsible for the health benefits of that drink. Resveratrol is an antioxidant that occurs naturally in the skins of grapes.

It turns out that grapes produce most resveratrol when they grow under stressful conditions—when vines have to deal with low temperatures, lack of nutrients, or fungal infections, for example. Wines from New York have more of it than wines from California, because life in New York is tougher. It also turns out that many plants other than grapevines produce resveratrol under stress, and it is quite possible that this compound serves to activate protective responses in them analogous to those that occur in animals on calorie-restricted diets.

In any case, if you give resveratrol to yeast cells, they live much longer than normal, just as if you had starved them. It is possible that it would do the same for worms, mice, and us, with an emphasis on "possible." If it did, resveratrol would be the ultimate free lunch or, rather, free fast, providing all the benefits of caloric restriction while allowing you to both have and eat your cake.

Without much more evidence to support their case, resveratrol enthusiasts have leapt to just this conclusion. Some of them have invoked high consumption of red wine as the cause of longevity on the island of Sardinia. Others have rushed to market. A product called Longevinex is already for sale: a stabilized, encapsulated form of resveratrol, one "serving" of which is said to equal the health-protective effects of five to fifteen glasses of red wine.

And this brings us back to the exhibit hall in Las Vegas, where products and claims go far beyond the limits of scientific evidence.

I have no doubt that genes influence life span and am intrigued by the discoveries of genetic mechanisms that extend life and reduce risks of age-related diseases by slowing metabolism and enhancing the body's defenses. I also expect that it will one day be possible to influence those mechanisms, maybe by taking antiaging pills.

But not now. And even when the pills become available, they may turn out to have devastating side effects. An objective look at the gap between the promises and realities of gene therapy is not encouraging. Since the mid-1990s, countless researchers and front-page stories in the media have led us to believe that gene therapies are going to revolutionize medicine, end disease, and postpone death. Where are those therapies? How many biotech enterprises have gone belly-up in attempts to capitalize on telomerase and other antiaging products?

These are the hard facts: It is theoretically possible to extend the human life span, but no methods of doing so are currently available. We do not really even know if caloric restriction will do it for us.* Furthermore, it is unlikely that any such methods will become available in time for anyone reading this book to make use of them.

And if scientifically based antiaging medicine becomes a reality, would it be a good thing? Would you want to use it?

I made a friend at the Okinawa Longevity Conference: Fernando Torres-Gil, associate dean and professor at the School of Public Policy and Social Research at UCLA. He is a foremost expert on the sociology of aging, having studied the implications of aging societies in Latin America, California, Korea, and elsewhere. In numerous articles, testimony before Congress, and talks around the world, Professor Torres-Gil has asked uncomfortable questions and pointed out disturbing facts about our changing demographics, among them:

- What are the political and economic implications of the growing numbers of old people in societies?
- In the United States, the bulk of the older population is white and English speaking, while the younger population is diverse and full of immigrants; how will this increasing social stratification change our country?
- A demographically healthy society needs more people in the middle-age range, because this is the fraction that supports the rest through work and productivity. How will disproportionate aging affect the nation?

---

*Roy Walford, M.D., one of the best-known advocates of caloric restriction, was diagnosed with ALS in his late seventies. (He died in 2004.) ALS (amyotrophic lateral sclerosis) is a devastating degenerative condition of the nervous system and an age-related disease. Given the claimed benefits of caloric restriction on brain health, one would not expect this result in one of its most diligent practitioners.

- What happens to caregiving in an aging society as more people require it but fewer women are available to provide it, because more of them have entered the workforce?
- What happens to retirement when Americans are no longer saving and are both retiring earlier (the average age is now sixty-three) and living longer?

Already in Japan, where the graying of society is more advanced, the economic and political effects of the demographic change are causing great social strain. It is unclear whether the Japanese system of national health insurance will be able to survive, just as it is unclear here whether Social Security as presently constituted will be able to handle so many people living far beyond the age of sixty-five.

These are just a few of the concerns facing a society where its oldest citizens are the fastest-growing segment of the population. And this is without considering the advent of interventions to extend human life. If effective antiaging medicine becomes available, it is sure to be expensive. Who will be able to afford it? Not the diverse population of non-English-speaking immigrants. It will be medicine for the rich, further hardening lines of social stratification and intensifying generational conflict.

What about on the personal level? A recent article by Susan Dominus in the *New York Times Magazine* titled "Life in the Age of Old, Old Age" looked at living examples and the problems they encounter. "Bill is 73, but his dad won't let him retire. Charlotte is 97, and her big sister still wants to tell her what to do. Natalie has been trying to please her mother since the Hoover administration." The article notes that "the philosophical impact on family dynamics will be profound, as parents continue to lean on children long past retirement themselves and people in their eighties learn what it means, at that age, to still be somebody's child." One of the people interviewed was Diana, a 102-year-old, who lives near her 74-year-old daughter. The daughter takes care of the mother and has done so for more than fifty years, ever since her father died. Diana recalled a doctor's telling her—when she was in her midsixties—that she would probably live to 100:

> Don't wish that on me, I told him. . . . All those people who want to live to 100—what's so good about it? Tell me—why do they think it's so great? I feel alone, I can't go to the store myself. I'm a burden. No, I don't think I'm happy I've lived so long. As for people in their thirties who think they'd like to live that long—don't they realize the world is just getting worse and worse? Don't they read the papers? I don't think you're going to like it here when you're 100. . . .The world is going to be upside down. . . . Ninety. . . . That's a good age. That's old enough.

You are going to hear more and more about antiaging medicine and life extension in the coming years. My bottom line for the here and now is that these theoretical breakthroughs serve only as serious distractions from what's important, namely, learning to accept the universality and inevitability of aging, understanding both its challenges and promises, and knowing how to keep minds and bodies as healthy as possible as we move through life's successive stages.

By the way, I returned to Las Vegas at the end of October 2004 to give a keynote talk at the first Primedia-sponsored, more scientific alternative to the A4M Conference. The event was titled "Integrative Medical Therapeutics for Anti-Aging Conference & Exposition." The plenary sessions were held in a room less than a quarter the size of A4M's venue, and, at least for the opening talks, more than half the seats were empty. For now, evidence-based antiaging medicine does not sell as well as hype.

4

WHY WE AGE

Aging is a deteriorative process, as most people should know. . . . The fact is that everything will [age], whatever the hell you do. Everything in the universe ages.

—Leonard Hayflick

There are many theories as to why we age. Some focus on the accumulation of errors in the genetic code, others invoke loss of telomeres. You don't need to know the details of all of these theories, but I thought it might be interesting to review two of them to give you a sense of the ways researchers are thinking. The first has to do with a chemical process called caramelization, and the second concerns oxidative stress. Both have practical import, the former because it suggests that dietary changes may reduce the risks of age-related diseases, the latter because it raises questions about whether we should take antioxidant vitamins and minerals in order to preserve youthful health and function as long as possible. Both theories suggest that senescence and longevity are separable, that age-related disease is not a necessary consequence of aging.

If you heat sugar in a pan, it first melts and then, when it reaches 170°C (338°F), it begins to turn brown, a change that happens faster in the presence of an acid catalyst, like a bit of lemon juice or vinegar. This process is called caramelization and is known to all experienced cooks. Although it looks simple, the chemical change, which involves the internal rearrangement of sugar molecules, is so complex that it is not fully understood. To give you just a hint of that complexity, let me share a section of a technical paper:

> Caramelization occurs in a sequence of six steps: The initial enolization reaction is of particular importance because it initiates the subsequent chain of events. These reactions give rise to aliphatic sugar degradation products which can react further to produce oxygen heterocyclic and carbocyclic compounds via aldol condensation.

I hope you will not be disappointed if I omit steps two through six.

Cooks need not understand the chemistry of caramelization in order to take advantage of it. They use a related process when they boil mixtures of sugar, cream, corn syrup, and butter to make caramel candy. In this case, the brown color and flavors result from a reaction between the sugars and the protein molecules in the cream and butter. It is called the Maillard reaction, after Louis-Camille Maillard, the French scientist who first described it in 1912. Also called the "browning reaction," this interaction of proteins and sugars is the basis of many appealing recipes. It is why roasts brown in the oven, why french frying turns potatoes crispy and tasty, why toast toasts, and why baked lasagna develops a delicious, chewy, golden-brown crust.

As with the caramelization of sugars, details of Maillard reactions are dauntingly complex, even for chemists. What is clear is that these chemical interactions not only explain the appearance, aroma, and flavor of many favorite foods but also account for a great many other phenomena, from the yellowing of old photographs made with egg-white emulsions to the brown color of soil (from combinations of sugars and proteins in decaying organic matter). Maillard had a sense of the vast reach of his discovery when he wrote in his original paper, "The implications of these facts seem to me as numerous as they are interesting in many branches of science." He specified human pathology as one of those branches.

Both the browning reaction and caramelization occur normally in living systems. They do not require the heat of an oven or saucepan; body temperature is perfectly con-ducive to them if chemical catalysts are present. Our bodies are full of sugars, proteins, and plenty of catalysts. Some bodies have more sugar circulating around them than oth-ers. Diabetics, especially, have intermittently high levels of blood sugar (glucose) when there is not enough insulin (or receptors for it) to facilitate sugar transport into cells. Doc-tors have long observed accelerated development of a num-ber of age-related diseases in people with diabetes, including cataracts and atherosclerosis. They also recognize that much of this pathology is the result of chemical reactions between glucose and proteins, a process called *glycation* that is noth-ing other than a Maillard reaction.

Think for a moment about caramel candy and that top layer of baked lasagna. Products of Maillard reactions tend to be brown and sticky. Glycation and related chemical reactions produce, for lack of a better word, gunk, and gunk gums up the works. Might aging be the result of the slow browning and caramelization of our tissues?*

Dr. Anthony Cerami, a medical researcher and inventor and member of the National Academy of Sciences, advanced just such a "glycation theory of aging" in 1985. It postulates that reactions between proteins and sugars in the body eventually form a class of compounds called "advanced glycation end products," or AGEs for short. AGEs can damage other proteins as well as DNA and RNA. They do so by fostering abnormal bonds between adjacent protein strands, a change called "cross-linking." Cross-linked proteins are deformed—less elastic, less flexible, and less able to perform their normal functions. It is cross-linking that makes the proteins in the lens of the eye turn opaque to form a cataract. Cross-linked proteins account for the wrinkling and sagging of old skin. Cross-linked proteins in blood vessels are the basis of arteriosclerosis, hardening of the arteries. Cross-linked proteins in the brain may contribute to the development of neurogenerative diseases like ALS, Parkinson's, and Alzheimer's.

Moreover, both AGEs and cross-linked proteins can initiate inflammatory and autoimmune responses and stimulate cells to proliferate, all of which can lead to further damage.

---

*Practitioners of Ayurveda, the traditional medicine of India, will find in these speculations echoes of their own theory of the causation of illness. Ayurvedic philosophy attributes illness to the accumulation of *ama*, toxic sludge thought to form from incompletely digested food. Many Ayurvedic treatments, like purging, vomiting, steam bathing, and oil massage, are intended to mobilize *ama* and help the body eliminate it.

In fact, many progressive diseases of aging can reasonably be attributed to the gradual accumulation of these substances and the changes they bring about in body structures and functions. The list includes hypertension, kidney disease, retinopathy, osteoarthritis, and, of course, all the complications of diabetes. These types of things happen in all of us but happen less quickly because there is less free sugar in the system than in the case of diabetics.

A promising area of drug development focuses on crosslink breakers, compounds that can undo the pathological bonds created in proteins by AGEs. Aspirin may be such a compound, and that property may explain some of its longterm health benefits, including reduced risk of cataracts and certain cancers. A more powerful cross-link breaker, pimagedine, is currently in clinical trials as a new treatment for diabetic nephropathy, the chronic kidney disease that is often a complication of diabetes.

A biogerontologist I know dismisses the whole "caramelization thing," as he puts it. It is, after all, just a theory. But what might be the practical recommendations that follow from a glycation theory of aging?

Because sugar in the body is mostly a product of carbohydrate metabolism and because it is the function of insulin to clear sugar from the blood, it would seem important to do whatever we can to keep metabolism fine tuned and insulin sensitivity high. The current obesity epidemic is forcing doctors to think about these issues, especially with the growing popularity of low-carbohydrate diets. In the wake of the epidemic obesity in children, we are also starting to see a dramatic increase in type 2 diabetes, the much more common type that used to be called adult-onset diabetes, now an inappropriate name when so many youngsters are being diagnosed with it. In type 2 diabetes, the pancreas produces enough insulin, but cells fail to respond to it. This loss of insulin sensitivity or, if you wish, the development of insulin resistance, represents loss of receptors for insulin on the surfaces of cells, a process that is influenced by both genes and lifestyle.

The genes responsible for insulin resistance—"thrifty genes," as they are sometimes called—are very common in our population because they were selected for by evolution when food was scarce and most people lived near starvation most of the time. If you are frequently on the edge of starvation, loss of sensitivity to insulin is a survival advantage; it allows you to take better advantage of calories when they are available and store them up as fat more efficiently. Stored fat gets you through times of scarcity. But now that we have food available all the time and in overabundance, those same genes become very disadvantageous. They can produce a spectrum of "metabolic syndromes," ranging from obesity to unhealthy patterns of fat and cholesterol in the blood to full-blown type 2 diabetes requiring drug treatment.

In addition to creating an overabundance of food in modern society, we have also changed the nature of many foods, refining and processing them from their natural state into forms that interact with our systems in new ways. This is most problematical with carbohydrate foods. Instead of eating our grains in whole form—parched, boiled, or chopped and cooked into chewy, chunky porridges—we mill them into flour, discarding the fibrous hull and oil-rich germ. This pulverized starch is digested very rapidly, causing spikes in blood sugar and corresponding surges in insulin secretion that, over time, lead to loss of sensitivity to that hormone in those with thrifty genes. It doesn't matter whether the flour is baked into white bread, "whole wheat" bread, pretzels,

chips, crackers, cookies, or pizza crusts; it's all finely pulverized starch with an enormous surface area for digestive
enzymes to work on, and it all rapidly converts to blood
sugar. And, of course, our diets are now flooded with sugar
itself, something the pancreases of our distant ancestors
never had to deal with. They got sugar only in ripe fruit and
an occasional honeycomb. We get it in almost every meal,
especially in foods and drinks flavored with cheap sweeten-
ers made from corn. This dietary change favors glycation
and the formation of AGEs.

I am not a proponent of the Atkins diet, but I think we
have to thank Dr. Atkins for drawing attention to the role of
carbohydrates in obesity. For years, conventional doctors
have focused obsessively on fat as the chief dietary culprit.
They have told us to cut fat consumption drastically and
have put countless people on low-fat diets without any
regard for the amount and kinds of carbohydrate foods they
were eating. At the same time, food manufacturers jumped
on the low-fat bandwagon, flooding the market with nonfat
and reduced-fat products. And all the while we have gotten
fatter and fatter.

Finally, there is the dawning of awareness among
physicians and dietitians that there are good and bad carbohydrates, just as there are good and bad fats. Bad carbohydrates are the refined, quickly digested ones that place a high
glycemic load on the system. (I'll give you specific dietary
advice later.)

Not only genes and diet affect insulin sensitivity and our
ability to process carbohydrates. Physical activity plays an
important role as well. Some people with type 2 diabetes are
able to put the disease in remission and avoid the need for

medication just by exercising vigorously and regularly, without changing how they eat. And some dietary supplements can help restore insulin sensitivity as well, among them chromium and alpha-lipoic acid. (Again, I'll give you detailed recommendations later.)

Consider these few facts:

- High levels of sugar in blood, even if transient, favor glycation and the production of compounds (AGEs) that damage body structures and distort its functions. This is true in everyone, regardless of genetic constitution.
- This damage and distortion, over time, are the probable basis of many chronic, degenerative diseases that increase in frequency the longer we live: age-related diseases, in other words.
- In people with thrifty genes—and that is a lot of us*—episodes of high blood sugar, when glycation reactions can occur, will be more frequent and will last longer, especially with the progressive loss of sensitivity to insulin.
- Even genetically susceptible people can minimize these problems by reducing the percentage of carbohydrate calories in the diet, by reducing or eliminating consumption of the kinds of carbohydrate foods that produce rapid increases in blood sugar, and by maintaining insulin sensitivity with exercise.

---

*It is a mistake to think that thrifty genes are unique to certain ethnic groups such as Native Americans, Hawaiians, Ashkenazic Jews, Gypsies, and others with high rates of type 2 diabetes. We do see the effects of these genes in populations that have been eating too much food and too much refined food for some time. But the recent appearance of obesity and type 2 diabetes in China and Japan, where the change to modern Western diets has come much more recently, suggests that these genotypes are more universal.

- In many ways, type 2 diabetes provides a model of accelerated aging, or at least of accelerated development of age-related disease. It is also the end point of a spectrum of metabolic problems that affect many more of us than those who will become diabetic.

Most health professionals who are informed about carbohydrate metabolism, metabolic syndromes, and insulin resistance are concerned about risks of obesity, cardiovascular disease, and diabetes. They are not yet aware of the "caramelization thing" and its relationship to the degenerative changes of aging. To my mind, this is an important area of research.

Before I leave the subject, I want to write briefly about another variety of gunk that is not the product of a Maillard reaction but rather represents the accumulation of cellular garbage. You know those "age spots" that most people develop and that doctors tell us have no significance? Actually, they may have a great deal of significance, because the same material that composes them gets deposited in many places that are not visible, including the brain. The name of this brown age pigment is *lipofuscin,* derived from the Greek root for "fat" and the Latin root for "dusky" or "dark." The term is inaccurate, at least the "fat" part. Lipofuscin is not one substance but a heterogeneous mixture of fats, proteins, and metals, especially iron. It is waste material, the consolidated debris of worn-out cellular structures that cannot be eliminated easily from the body, and it piles up inside cells, particularly ones that are no longer actively dividing. That includes heart muscle cells and nerve cells.

Clearly, lipofuscin is a marker of age. It starts to accumulate right after birth and continues to do so throughout life at an accelerating rate. We still don't know whether it is a cause of aging or a result of it, or whether cells stuffed full of it suffer damage from it. Evidence on these points is contradictory, and scientific opinion is divided. Most of our knowledge of how lipofuscin accumulates comes from studies of the eye. A layer of cells behind the retina is very rich in it, more so in people over forty. Those cells are responsible for providing nutrients and removing wastes from the light-sensitive cells of the retina, and some researchers think lipofuscin impairs their functioning. That could cause aging of the eye and age-related macular degeneration, one of the main causes of loss of vision in the elderly. (A routine eye examination can show how much age pigment is present.)

Other experts think that lipofuscin is a product of the interaction of cellular waste with free radicals, the highly reactive molecules generated by damaging oxidation reactions (more on this in a moment). It is also possible that when large amounts of age pigment are packed into cells, the cells become more susceptible to oxidative stress.

That leads to a much more important topic, the free radical theory of aging, which is all about oxidative stress and is so prominent in scientific thinking that it is essential for you to understand its general outlines.

Oxidation is the chemist's term for the process of removing electrons from an atom or molecule. Oxygen happens to be particularly good at stripping electrons from other atoms and molecules and so has lent its name to the general process. In other words, oxygen is a good oxidizing agent, but so are other substances (chlorine, for one). Oxygen itself is caustic and destructive; you can see that in the oxidation, or rusting, of iron, when it turns a solid metal into a flaky, corroded material.* We need oxygen to live, but high concentrations of it are toxic to living things.

When oxygen and other oxidizing agents strip electrons away from organic molecules—the large ones that living systems depend on—they can actually shred those molecules, rendering them defective or useless. Therefore, living systems must have defenses against oxygen and oxidation in order to protect their constituents from damage.

Those defenses may have originally evolved for a different purpose: as protection against solar radiation, which was much more intense in the early history of our planet. When radiation interacts with water, it splits it, producing oxygen and, along the way, a series of unstable intermediates called *free radicals*. Free radicals exist independently—very briefly, in some cases—and are distinguished by an unstable electronic configuration: an unpaired electron. In an effort to achieve stability, free radicals react with any molecules they meet, stripping electrons from them. This creates more unstable molecules that then attack their neighbors in falling-domino-like chain reactions. The only ways these reactions stop are when two radicals react with each other in such a way as to form a stable molecule or when the reaction products are too weak to interact with other molecules.

By the time a free-radical chain reaction fizzles out, it may have ripped through vital components of cells like a tornado, causing extensive damage. In fact, this is exactly the

---

*The opposite of oxidation is *reduction,* the addition of electrons, a confusing term because it suggests that something has been lost rather than gained. A mnemonic device that has helped chemistry students get the two opposed processes straight is "LEO the Lion says GER"—that is, Loss of Electrons is Oxidation, Gain of Electrons is Reduction.

mechanism of radiation poisoning. Exposure to radiation, whether from X-rays or nuclear explosions, breaks down water in our bodies, generating free radicals that damage DNA, proteins, cell membranes, and other vital structures. The symptoms of radiation poisoning—immediate gastro-intestinal havoc, later loss of hair, and, much later, development of bone cancer and leukemia—are consequences of that free-radical damage.

Green plants also split water and generate oxygen in a more controlled fashion, using the energy of the sun. This is photosynthesis, which enables plants to capture solar energy and make simple sugar (glucose) from carbon dioxide in the air. And both plants and animals reverse this process during *respiration,* when they metabolize (burn) glucose with oxygen, producing water and carbon dioxide. In all these bio-chemical pathways, the same highly reactive intermediates are generated as in the interactions of radiation with water in nonliving systems. As a class, these dangerous molecules are often called *reactive oxygen species,* or ROS. Two of them are free radicals (the hydroxyl radical and the super-oxide radical); the third is hydrogen peroxide, the familiar bleach and disinfectant that destroys colors and kills germs by its oxidizing action.

Scientists tell us that life began in the oceans when very little oxygen was present in the earth's atmosphere and solar radiation was much more intense because there was no ozone layer to screen it out. The earliest life did not depend on oxygen, but when ancient bacteria first developed the ability to photosynthesize, they were protected from the dangerous products of their own biochemistry by defensive systems that were already in place, having evolved to protect their ancestors from radiation. Those *antioxidant defenses* were inherited by all later life-forms and made it possible for cells to photosynthesize and respire, despite the toxic products of those innovations and an increasing concentration of oxygen in the air (the result of photosynthesis on an ever-widening scale).

I don't want to drive you away with chemistry. For those who want more detail on the nature of oxygen, oxidation, and the free radical theory of aging, I cannot recommend too highly the book *Oxygen: The Molecule That Made the World* by Nick Lane, a London-based biochemist and science writer. I am in total agreement with Lane's presentation of the theory and with his further speculations about the centrality of oxidative stress to the development of age-related diseases. I have drawn on many of his ideas in this section.

Oxidative stress is simply the total burden placed on organisms by the constant production of free radicals in the normal course of metabolism, added to whatever oxidative pressures come from the environment. The latter include natural and artificial radiation; toxins in air, food, and water; and miscellaneous sources of oxidizing activity, such as tobacco smoke, one of the most concentrated delivery systems of free radicals.

Here is the minimum amount of chemistry you need to keep in mind in order to understand the implications for aging and ways to moderate its less welcome effects:

Oxygen is corrosive and toxic to living things. We obtain energy by burning fuel—that is, by combining digested food with oxygen from the air we breathe in a metabolic process that generates the same dangerous reactive oxygen species that account for the harmfulness of radiation. These species include powerful oxidizing agents and free radicals that can initiate destructive chain reactions in cellular structures. In addition, we are exposed to environmental sources of free radicals. Our bodies are equipped with antioxidant defenses as protection against these dangers. They include physical barriers to contain free radicals at their sites of production within cells; enzymes that neutralize ROS; substances derived from the diet (like vitamins C and E) that can "quench" free radicals by donating electrons to them, stopping free-radical chain reactions early in their course; repair mechanisms to take care of oxidative damage to DNA, proteins, and membranes; and complex stress responses that range from programmed cell suicide if damage is too great to the activation of master control genes that regulate metabolism and defensiveness.

A good case can be made that health depends on a balance between oxidative stress and antioxidant defenses. Senescence and the appearance of age-related diseases represent the inability of antioxidant defenses to cope with oxidative stress over time with the steady accumulation of defects in DNA, in proteins, and in membranes. From this point of view, "senescence" and "longevity" are not synonymous. If antioxidant defenses are strong, long life without disease should be possible. Certainly, this is the case with some centenarians, who enjoy good health until near the end, then decline rapidly. Most people would like to age that way, and if more of us could do it, we might not have to worry so much about the economic consequences of greater longevity. If the oldest old were to remain relatively disease free, their impact on the health-care system might not be so great, even if there were many more of them in a population.

As I write, I am picturing in my mind a ninety-two-year-old woman I met two days ago at an academic conference in Wisconsin. I would have guessed her age at seventy, basing that on her energy as well as her appearance. There was a great discrepancy between her chronological age and her apparent age, or, as some would say, her biological age. Probably she enjoys the protective effects of unusually efficient antioxidant defenses. Very likely, differing efficiency of those defenses explains why some of my high school classmates at the reunion I mentioned earlier appeared hardly to have aged, while others seemed much older than their years.

The pattern of a long, disease-free life is exactly what we see in animals on caloric restriction and in worms and insects with genetically engineered longevity. Recall that the mechanisms responsible for the beneficial effects of these interventions involve master control genes that slow metabolism and activate stress responses that are part of the antioxidant defense system. With slower metabolism, there is less oxidative stress and reduced production of free radicals. This, in turn, reduces the formation of advanced glycation end products (AGEs), which form in the presence of free radicals and exert their toxic effects by generating more free radicals and causing more oxidative damage. It also reduces the accumulation of lipofuscin, which appears to form when cellular debris reacts with free radicals.

If health is dependent on the efficiency of our antioxidant defenses, especially in older age, what can we do to maintain them? If you look at the various classes of defenses listed above, the one that seems most under our control is "substances derived from the diet." Those substances include vitamins, minerals, protective compounds (phytonutrients), and even some toxins, all of plant origin. So the most practical step we can take to defend ourselves against the ravages of oxidative stress is to *eat more plants*. In a later chapter, I will go into detail about the kinds and amounts of plants we should be eating. Here I will just say that most people I meet are not eating the quantity or variety of plant-based foods they should be—not even close to what Okinawans eat, for example. I will also note that many natural toxins—both those that occur in culinary herbs and spices and those in the plant intoxicants that people consume throughout the world—may all help to bolster our defenses against oxidative stress. The latter category includes betel, qat, opium, coca, coffee, tea, chocolate, kava, and marijuana.

Much research focuses on the identification, isolation, and study of compounds of plant origin with antioxidant effects. A big, open question is whether we should supplement our diets with them.

Go into any health-food store, drugstore, or supermarket, and you will find a great many antioxidant supplements for sale, including vitamins C and E, beta-carotene, green-tea extracts, resveratrol, curcumin (from turmeric), and Pycnogenol (from the bark of a pine tree). Not only is there insufficient evidence that taking them will do you any good, some experts think they might be harmful. (I am not one of them. I continue to take a daily antioxidant formula and recommend it to others as well. I'll give it to you later on.)

Here are the arguments against taking these supplements:

First, there is a simple physical problem. Antioxidant compounds like vitamin C are needed in the liquid contents of cells, near the respiratory "factories"—the mitochondria—that spew out free radicals, but when you take them as supplements, they mostly stay in the bloodstream and extracellular fluid. This is less of a concern with vitamin E, which is fat soluble and acts mainly to protect the fatty layers of cell membranes from free-radical chain reactions, but it is a concern for most of the others.

Second, some of these compounds are able to function as pro-oxidants as well as antioxidants. Vitamin C is in this group. Under some circumstances it can accept electrons from another molecule rather than donate electrons to quench a free radical. If you flood the system with more vitamin C than you normally get from fruits and vegetables in the diet, you do not know which action will predominate. It would be most unwise to add to the body's oxidative stress by giving it dietary supplements it does not need or want.

And this possibility is of great practical concern. Not long ago, I and other doctors recommended taking supplemental beta-carotene, the most prominent member of the carotenoid family of plant pigments, in order to reduce cancer risks. Later research showed that smokers and ex-smokers who followed this advice seemed to be more likely to develop lung and colorectal cancers, apparently because beta-carotene acts as a pro-oxidant in them. We knew that fruits and vegetables containing beta-carotene are highly protective against cancer in general. We assumed that daily capsules of beta-carotene would be a convenient way for more people to take advantage of that protection. We were wrong—at least when it comes to smokers and ex-smokers. Why?

One theory is that beta-carotene becomes a pro-oxidant when it is removed from the context in which nature produces it—that is, as a member of a large family of red, yellow, and orange pigments that always occur together in brightly colored fruits (like tomatoes and cantaloupes) and vegetables (carrots, ripe bell peppers), including dark, leafy greens (where they are masked by chlorophyll). As a family, these compounds are important components of the antioxidant defenses of plants. They work in us, too, but we cannot produce them in our bodies and and so must get them by eating plants. Other carotenoids include alpha-carotene, lutein (which protects the eyes from cataracts and macular degeneration), lycopene (which reduces risk of prostate cancer), phytoene, and zeaxanthin. I now recommend only supplements that contain a balanced mix of carotenoids, but I tell people that even these may not be equivalent to the fruits and vegetables that contain them.

Another possibility is that whether beta-carotene inhibits cancer or promotes it has to do with the context in which it is placed rather than that from which it is taken. In other words, something about the biochemical state of the cells of tobacco smokers might determine which action predominates, pro-oxidant or antioxidant. If that is so, it would raise further questions about when and how to take antioxidant supplements to get the desired effect, questions we cannot now answer with certainty.

The final argument against adding these compounds to the diet is the most thought provoking of all. Up to now, I have painted oxidative stress as all bad, a negative force that damages the structures and impairs the functions of life and accelerates the development of age-related disease. But, in fact, oxidative stress, including free radicals, has another face, because the body relies on it for protection against other kinds of disease, especially infectious disease. Infection increases oxidative stress. And that rise in oxidative stress signals genes to activate the immune system in order to deal with germs.

One key result of that activation is the inflammatory response, marked by localized redness, heat, swelling, and pain at the site of infection. These changes represent an influx of blood and immune cells to the site, and while they may be uncomfortable, they are absolutely necessary. Inflammation itself has two faces, one positive, one negative. It is a cornerstone of the body's defenses against infection and a crucial part of the healing system; yet it can also cause disease on its own, as in autoimmunity. Because inflammation can turn against the body, it must stay where it is supposed to stay and end when it is supposed to end. It is, therefore, tightly regulated by an intricate system of hormones, some of which intensify (upregulate) it while others mute (downregulate) it. Health depends on a dynamic balance of those opposing pressures. If inflammation is too little and too late, germs can get the upper hand; if it is too much and too long or if it occurs when it is not needed, other types of disease result.

If antioxidant supplements really do reduce oxidative stress, then they might weaken needed immune responses to infection by blocking the very signal that tells the immune system to mount a defensive response. (This is analogous to the argument for not giving aspirin to people with ordinary fevers. Elevation of body temperature is an immune response that favors the efficiency of cells that fight germs; lowering it artificially makes it harder for those cells to do their job.)

I am not too concerned about this last possibility, because I am in awe of the body's ability to maintain homeostasis—that is, to maintain the equilibrium it wants despite most forces that impinge on it. Here is an example of what I mean. I meet many people, including some practitioners of natural and alternative medicine, who worry unduly about the body's acid/alkaline balance, its pH. They test the pH of their saliva regularly (with paper test strips) and tell everyone to follow an "alkalinizing diet," meaning few or no animal products, no refined sugar, and no white flour. This may be good dietary advice for other reasons, but it has nothing to do with the acidity or alkalinity of our blood and tissue fluids. Nor is salivary pH an indicator of those values. Because pH is such an important determinant of basic biochemistry and physiology, including the function of nerve and muscle cells, the body cannot afford to take chances with it. The body's homeostatic mechanisms keep pH constant through a wide range of external changes, including the varying nature of what you eat and drink. If you drink a glass of lemon juice, it may erode your dental enamel and will probably irritate the lining of your esophagus, but it will not change your body's pH one whit.

In the same way, because reliance on rising oxidative stress as a signal for immune activity against infection is so vital to survival, I suspect the body is perfectly capable of ignoring, neutralizing, or otherwise managing the perturbing influence of an extra helping or two of dietary antioxidants, whether in carrots or in capsules.

There are some other important implications of the fact that oxidative stress is useful to the body in some circumstances. Infection is a major source of this kind of stress in early life and has the potential to kill individuals before they reach reproductive age. It is likely, therefore, that natural selection favored the evolution of a defensive system that responded to oxidative stress and even came to depend on it as a signal to spring into action—by mounting an inflammatory response, for example. When the immune system defeats an infectious assault, oxidative stress drops and the defensive system calms down. In such cases, the cause of rising oxidative stress is external to the body and the body can eliminate it.

This is a clever strategy for defense against a common threat to survival in early life, but we may pay a high price for it in later life when we advance past our reproductive years. As we age, rising oxidative stress is a consequence of depending on oxygen to obtain energy. For example, the mitochondria in our cells, where respiration occurs, lose their integrity and leak more free radicals. This elicits the same response as infection does, but now the inflammation and other defensive actions that occur serve no purpose and cause damage rather than healing. This source of rising oxidative stress cannot be eliminated.

In recent years, scientists have begun to recognize that misplaced, unnecessary, and prolonged inflammation may be a common root of many chronic, degenerative diseases that until now have appeared to have nothing in common. Cardiologists agree that coronary heart disease and atherosclerosis begin as an inflammatory process in the lining of arteries. Alzheimer's disease begins as inflammation in the brain. In all the autoimmune diseases, like rheumatoid arthritis and lupus, the damage to tissues and organs is the result of inappropriate inflammation. Rheumatoid arthritis is more common in young people, but most of these inflammatory disorders become more prominent with age; in fact, they account for much of the age-related disease we would like to prevent.

Clearly, oxidative stress has two faces: it may be useful to the body early in life to call forth defensive action against external threats to health, but it becomes increasingly harmful as we age, by continuously activating those defenses when they are not needed, causing damaging inflammation. Nick Lane and others call this scheme the "double-agent" theory of aging. Lane writes: "Because oxidative stress is pivotal to our recovery from infections in youth, and therefore affects our likelihood of surviving to have children, it is positively selected for by natural selection to our own detriment in old age."

This idea is sensible, but I am not sure it is the ultimate answer to the question of why we age. Everything I have written about here describes changes associated with aging, such as the caramelization of our proteins and sugars with the production of damaging age-related glycation end products, or the accumulation of lipofuscin in cells, or the toxic effects of oxidative stress. But why do these changes happen? Why, for instance, do old mitochondria become leaky, allowing more free radicals to escape and trigger inappropriate inflammation?

The best answer to these questions is suggested in Leonard Hayflick's quote at the beginning of this chapter: "Everything in the universe ages." Consider that statement for a moment.

A favorite tree near my house is now senescent. It is a perfectly shaped Arizona cypress *(Cupressus arizonica)*, almost sixty feet tall, a very drought-tolerant evergreen with blue-green leaves and a symmetrical form that tree experts call "pyramidal" or "steeple-shaped." Last year, its top began to turn brown and die back. A tree expert diagnosed the problem as crown canker, a fungal disease. He treated my tree, but this spring, the dieback was worse, and I learned that the real problem is that my tree is old, probably sixty years old or more, which is about the maximum life span of an Arizona cypress. Crown canker is an opportunistic infection that strikes susceptible hosts. Old age has weakened my tree, and it now has an age-related disease that will probably kill it.

The Grenville Mountains once stretched from Greenland across Quebec and Ontario and into the United States and were as high as the Himalayas. Created by the collision of protocontinents, they are long gone, worn down by erosion, covered by ocean sediments, the rocks that composed them recycled by advancing and retreating ice sheets into the Laurentians, a low range in southern Quebec, now a popular recreation area for residents of Montreal and Ottawa. The Grenville Mountains aged and passed away. Their "bones"—the rocks that make up the Laurentians—are old rocks.

Look up in the night sky at the familiar constellation of Orion the Hunter. The bright, reddish star in the upper left corner is Betelgeuse, a red supergiant, which would engulf the earth if it were to replace our sun. It is an old star, having left the long, stable period of middle age that astrophysicists call the "main sequence" of stellar evolution. Stars in the main sequence, like our sun, fuse hydrogen to helium by nuclear reactions that generate enough energy to balance the inward collapse of gravity. This state of equilibrium results from the balanced tension of two opposing forces, much as health results from the balance between oxidative stress and anti-oxidant defenses. But sooner or later, as in the case of Betelgeuse, hydrogen fuel runs out, other nuclear reactions begin in order to stave off gravitational collapse, and the star leaves the main sequence on a path that leads first to cooling and expansion, then to contraction, sometimes to catastrophic collapse, and eventually to the formation of a stellar "corpse," a tiny, inert remnant of a once brilliant star.

It is easy to distinguish old trees from young trees, old mountains from young mountains, old stars from young stars. And no one has any difficulty recognizing an old person. Everything in the universe ages, although different things may do it in different ways and on vastly different time scales. Nothing is immune to the changes that time brings. Moreover, time points in one direction.

I remember as a teenager making a very short, odd film with a home movie camera, using a technique I discovered in a photography magazine. I filmed a friend sitting outdoors in a chair reading a newspaper, then tearing the newspaper up and throwing handfuls of it to the wind until it was all gone. The trick was to hold the camera upside down and film the sequence in slow motion. Then, when the developed film came back, I cut the sequence out and reversed it on the reel of the projector, so that the end was now the beginning. The effect on screen was that a person sitting calmly in a chair reaches up and begins catching pieces of paper that blow toward him. The pieces come together, one by one, until they form a complete newspaper, which he then reads.

Of course, this bit of trick photography depicts what could never happen. We commonly see order breaking down into disorder, but we do not observe disorder spontaneously giving rise to order. Nor do we see old trees turn into young trees or senescent red supergiant stars evolve into hot, young, blue-white stars. And we never observe people growing younger.

This directionality of evolutionary change has been called "time's arrow," a nickname for the Second Law of Thermodynamics. That law states simply that while the energy of the universe remains constant, its disorder or randomness constantly increases. We are subject to the Second Law of Thermodynamics, as are all things living and nonliving, and our aging is an expression of increasing disorder in our bodies with the passage of time. That is why old mitochondria lose their integrity and leak more free radicals into our cells. It is why we will never be able to reverse the aging process. It is why the concept of antiaging medicine is wrong from the start.

So please forget about antiaging and avoid obsession with life extension. Instead, let's focus on preventing or minimizing the impact of age-related disease, on separating longevity and senescence, on learning how to live long and well, on how to age gracefully.

5

THE DENIAL OF AGING

I think like a young person and, although I try to keep myself fit and active, I won't be taking desperate measures like face-lifts and plastic surgery. I'm a great believer in letting nature take its course and living with what I've been given.

—Sharon Stone

With mirth and laughter let old wrinkles come.

—Shakespeare, *The Merchant of Venice*

If aging is written into the laws of the universe, then acceptance of it must be a prerequisite for doing it in a graceful way. Yet nonacceptance of aging seems to be the rule in our society, not the exception. A great many people try to deny its reality and progress. Two of the most obvious ways of doing so are the use of cosmetics products and cosmetic surgery. I will mention others but would like to examine these two in a bit of detail.

Up to now, I have reviewed for you the science of aging,

given you my thoughts on life extension and antiaging medicine, and urged you to concentrate on separating longevity and senescence. I have suggested that the most important goal is to learn how to reduce the risks of age-related disease in order to enjoy health into advanced years. Before I tell you what I know about that subject, I would like you to think about both the positive and negative aspects of aging. Many people think only of the latter and never consider the former. The motivation to deny aging is rooted in that skewed perception.

In the next chapter, I write about the positive changes that aging can bring, I hope in a new and useful way. In this chapter I want to look squarely at the negatives, which are uppermost in so many minds. Here is a list of words people commonly equate with "old":

> ancient
> antediluvian
> antiquated
> antique
> archaic
> brittle
> bygone
> dated
> decayed
> decrepit
> dowdy
> dried-up
> dry
> dusty
> elderly
> enduring
> faded

frail
fusty
gray
grizzled
hoary
lasting
long-lived
mature
passé
seasoned
senile
shriveled
stale
superannuated
timeworn
tough
used up
useless
venerable
veteran
vintage
weathered
wise
withered
worthless
wrinkled
yellowed

When I look over this list, I find only a few qualities I would call positive or attractive: "enduring," "lasting," "mature," "seasoned," "venerable," "veteran," "vintage," and "wise." "Enduring" and "lasting" suggest strength through continuity; the former derives from the Latin root for "hard," closely relating it to "tough" farther down the list. Though "enduring" is a positive attribute, "old and tough" is not a particularly pleasing combination. The other positives revolve around a core sense of ripening with maturity, a key concept that I will return to in the following chapter. But although ripening can bring wisdom and fullness, "ripe" can easily connote "rotten" or "over the hill," which brings on the whole cascade of strong negatives in the list: "decayed," "decrepit," "dried-up," "dusty," "faded," "senile," "shriveled," "stale," "withered," "wrinkled," "yellowed," and these easily lead to "used up," "useless," and "worthless." Of all the word associations I have collected, it is this last one that bothers me most. Does the worth of human life diminish with age?

I'm afraid that in the judgment of many in our society, it does. Here is one bit of evidence from, of all places, the United States Environmental Protection Agency. In April 2003, the EPA proposed reducing the value of a senior citizen's life to 63 percent or less of the $6.1 million value per individual it uses when doing required cost-benefit analyses for environmental programs. (The effect of this devaluation would be to limit the reach of antipollution rules, a boon to industry.) Environmental politics aside, it is clear that ours is increasingly a youth-oriented culture. We value and celebrate the beauty and vigor of youth in fashion and entertainment. We do not celebrate the virtues of maturity. Too often the elderly are viewed as "old and gray and only in the way," in the words of an old song.

I do not think I need to belabor the point that more of us look at the negative aspects of aging than at the positives. There are real problems that aging brings—physical ones, such as aches and pains, decreased mobility, and diminished sensory acuity, and psychological ones, such as memory impairment, social isolation, and the loss of friends and family—but there are also strategies for managing them. Denial of aging is an obstacle to learning and implementing those strategies.

One of the most common ways to deny aging is to try to mask its outward signs. Look at the profusion of cosmetics products that claim to be age erasers and wrinkle removers. In some cases, there is no pretense that the creams and lotions are anything other than cover-ups; in other cases ads and labels actually suggest rejuvenating and age-reversing properties.

Human beings have been applying cosmetics since antiquity. Ancient Egyptians developed them into an art form and documented their use in both paintings and texts. In those sources I discern two facts that are just as relevant to contemporary society. The first is that cosmetics have always served two main purposes: enhancement of beauty and sexual attractiveness and the masking of age-related changes in visible parts of the body. The second is that women have always been the more dedicated users, because they are more likely to be judged and valued for their beauty and sexual attractiveness, which men tend to associate with youthfulness.

The use of cosmetics for beautification is outside the scope of this discussion. It is strongly influenced by cultural standards, and those vary greatly. In some cultures, body scarification and tattooing are ultimate beauty marks, for instance, while in others they are not. But I do want to talk about the use of cosmetics to cover up or try to undo the signs of aging.

The first thing to be said about products on today's market that claim to be anything other than masking agents is that most of them are bogus. Some of those products are phenomenally expensive, supposedly because they incorporate rare and exotic ingredients, and many invoke scientific research to explain how they rejuvenate the skin. Actually, this is no different from the false claims and lack of evidence for the antiaging technologies I wrote about earlier, except that in the case of cosmetics, the claims are even sillier, the lack of evidence more complete, and the price gouging more egregious.

Here is an excerpt from a *New York Times* article about a new wave of antiaging skin care products, beginning with a description of Re-Storation Deep Repair Facial Serum at $200 an ounce:

> Its ingredients include extracts from soybeans, kelp, lemon grass, and rose hips, and the antioxidants alpha-lipoic acid, green tea, and grapeseed extract. Its manufacturer is called Z. Bigatti, a name that might conjure images of Milanese scientists and laboratories in the Dolomites, even though its founder, Dr. Jennifer Biglow, is a dermatologist based in St. Paul, Minn., who speaks with an accent few would mistake for Continental.
>
> "My business partner made it up," Dr. Biglow said of the name. "I thought it was kind of sexy. It could be a car, it could be leather. It could be anything luxurious."
>
> Deep Repair Facial Serum is one of a new breed of radically priced so-called antiaging skin care concoctions that have made the legendarily expensive Crème de la Mer—at $90 an ounce—seem a meager extravagance. Earlier this year, for instance, the Swiss company La Prairie introduced Crème Cellulaire Radiance, which it says will improve skin's elasticity through a combination of plant-based estrogens derived from soybeans and wild yams, among other things. The cream costs $500

for a 1.7 ounce jar. It lists sixty-two ingredients on the side of the packaging, the first being water.

Also new to the counters of stores like Neiman Marcus is Intensité Crème Lustre at $375 for two ounces from Ré Vivé, a company started by a plastic surgeon named Gregory Bays Brown. (Ré Vivé "is just a contrived name, a bogus French name," Dr. Brown said from his office in Louisville, Ky.) The product is so costly, he said, because the primary ingredient is a protein called Insulin-like Growth Factor (IGF), which, he said, stimulates collagen production in order to plump up the skin and diminish the appearance of lines. IGF costs Dr. Brown $30,000 a gram, he said, with one gram enough to produce about 200,000 jars (which works out to 15 cents of IGF per $375 jar, but the company says hundreds of thousands of dollars of research went into IGF's formulation).

I am unconvinced that any of the ingredients in these expensive products has antiaging effects. There is ongoing scientific research on the topical application of antioxidants—vitamins C and E and green-tea extract, for example—to block and perhaps undo some of the skin damage caused by the sun's ultraviolet rays, but the result is not to make the skin younger. There are also very sensible ways to maintain natural skin health. They start with good nutrition, especially intake of adequate amounts of essential fatty acids (by supplementation, if you cannot get enough from your diet), as well as drinking enough water every day, avoiding excessive use of soaps and skin irritants, and, especially, protecting the skin from solar radiation, which has a cumulative effect. The extensive facial wrinkling of older Native Americans of the southwest deserts, where I live, is not a normal sign of aging. It represents sun damage over a lifetime and can be prevented. Integrative skin care also means applying safe and effective natural products with anti-inflammatory activity. (Such products are just coming to market.)

Wild yam extracts do nothing for the skin, topically or otherwise. The Mexican wild yam *(Dioscorea villosa)* contains a compound called diosgenin that is used by pharmaceutical chemists as a starting material to synthesize estrogenic hormones, but diosgenin itself is inactive in humans, and our bodies cannot convert it to anything with hormonal activity. As for applying IGF to the skin, it does not sound like a good idea to me, even if you have only fifteen cents' worth of it in your jar of antiaging cream. IGF is a known tumor promoter.

For those readers who use cosmetics, let me clarify my concerns. It is fine to use these products if you enjoy them, if they make you feel good, if you are using them to make yourself more beautiful and more attractive to your own eyes and to the eyes of others. I would ask you, however, to look carefully at your motivations and make sure they do not include a desire to undo the normal changes in appearance that aging brings. If that desire is present, you are vulnerable to the unfounded claims of manufacturers who want to take your money and to seduction by the fantasy that you can stop, slow, or reverse aging. That path leads away from acceptance of a natural and universal process central to our experience as human beings. Following it will make it harder for you to master the art of healthy aging.

Obviously, cosmetic surgery can be an even more powerful and costly seduction, not to mention a riskier one. Once available only to the most affluent, it has recently become much cheaper, much more mainstream, and much more widely practiced. More than 70 percent of those who opt for cosmetic surgery today earn less than $50,000 a year.

As with cosmetics, people resort to surgery to alter their appearance for very different reasons. When they do it to repair birth defects like harelips or damage from trauma, I have no quarrel with it. (That is properly called reconstructive rather than cosmetic surgery.) When young people get nose jobs or breast augmentations, I may consider their actions frivolous, but it is not of great concern to me unless the procedures pose significant risks to health. But when I see increasing numbers of older men and women getting face-lifts, Botox injections, and fat implantations to fill in wrinkles, I do worry.

We have all seen disastrous results of plastic surgery: procedures that did not heal or, more commonly, faces pulled so tight that their owners look like the Bride of Frankenstein. And these less appealing outcomes of surgical alteration of the face become more grotesque as people age. Of course, the procedures can be done skillfully and can give more pleasing results. So if cosmetic surgery makes people feel better about themselves, makes them feel more beautiful and attractive, and therefore gives them better quality of life and improves their relationships, again, it is probably not my place to argue against it. But I think it is a problem when their primary reason for having plastic surgery is to pretend that aging is not occurring.

Remember that your true age—your biological age—is determined not by years but by the state of your body's structure and functions. That probably has to do with the balance between oxidative stress and antioxidant defenses, with the accumulation of errors in the DNA of your cells, with the extent of caramelization that has occurred in your tissues, with the integrity of your mitochondria. In the words of a female plastic surgeon, "It happens one day. You're fine until a certain point because you can't see what happens inside your body, and then one day you see signs of aging in your face. It's a sharp reminder of mortality." Plastic surgery cannot fix what happens inside your body; it can only dull the sharpness of the reminder. And, to my mind, that is movement away from reality. I agree with Carl Jung, who wrote: "As a physician I am convinced that it is hygienic . . . to discover in death a goal toward which one can strive; and that shrinking away from it is something unhealthy and abnormal which robs the second half of life of its purpose." *Because aging reminds us of our mortality, it can be a primary stimulus to spiritual awakening and growth.*

The relative percentage of men seeking cosmetic surgery has not changed in the past twenty years, while that of women has skyrocketed. And women are undergoing it at ever-younger ages, often getting their eyes done before they reach forty.

"How is it really," asks Daphne Merkin, writing about the subject as her fiftieth birthday approaches, "that American women have been so successfully terrorized by the thought of showing their age—of becoming what even the fiercely independent-minded lesbian writer May Sarton described as 'an old woman, a grotesque miserable animal'—that they will spend enormous amounts of money and time in the effort to stave off a process that was once considered to be a natural, even revered one by any means, ranging from the patently ludicrous to the purportedly scientific to the bloodily effective?" She also includes this comment from a medical researcher at Columbia University: "Aging is nature's way of preparing us for death. That's why we hate old people."

I was surprised to hear that kind of hatred coming from a friend of mine, a woman only slightly younger than I, who teaches yoga, does grief counseling, is well read in the literature of many spiritual traditions, and is not afraid to talk about death and dying. I think of her as a wise elder or, at least, a person in the process of becoming one.

"I never admitted to myself how repelled I am by old people," she told me recently. "I was walking on the beach and saw an old couple coming toward me, maybe in their mideighties. They had their arms around each other, and I know I should have applauded the fact that they were out walking together and being affectionate, but all I could see was the sagging flesh, those wattles under the chin, and I had to look away. Then I had to face the degree of my antipathy toward them. I hate people who look that way. Their appearance repels me, especially their faces. This was a revelation for me, not a comfortable one."

I can find no explanation for her reaction other than the obvious one. She sees in these people what she will become, and she hates them for reminding her of it.

How commonly do the old have corresponding feelings of contempt for the young? "I suppose the one good thing to be said about having already aged is that it gives you the upper hand in a strange, secretive sort of way," says Merkin. "I mean, you can look at young girls in their barely-there whiffs of clothes—their abbreviated tank tops or skirts that stop just below the pelvis, strutting their juicy stuff, and think: Just you wait, just you wait. Your spring-chicken days are numbered, all you fine-feathered chickadees."

I've asked a number of my contemporaries about their denial of aging and their susceptibility or resistance to the temptations of products and procedures.

One woman friend, an art dealer in New York, now sixty, replied:

I feel that getting older is interesting—very. There are challenges that put you face to face with yourself and close-up! When I close my eyes and think about aging, I see myself quieter, sitting still and thinking deeply. This is the image that surfaces, and I am glad to see it, because it is a nice image. Aging means to me many different things: the physical diminishing, the morning stiffness, the wrinkles, my compromised knees. But aging also contains all the power all at once of the information I have gathered, powerful moments experienced.

I deny aging very little. How can I? It is what is so— one ages! Nonetheless I work my knees as if they were brand new, knowing they aren't. I had my first Botox injection—in order to look less worried, not younger. I haven't been tempted to do cosmetic surgery, because I know that it won't address the real issues, and I actually hate the masklike look that most face-lifts create. My friends try to talk me into it, and when they do, I think about it, but then a red light flashes in my mind's eye.

I try to accept changes in my appearance and in my body. Some of this is difficult and challenging for me. It is the limitation I feel in my degenerating knees that bothers me as much as the wrinkles in my face and the slight stoop I sometimes catch in the store window as I glimpse my image in passing. All the things I love to do most depend on my knees. The wrinkles won't interfere with my enjoyment of hiking, swimming, exercising, and being in nature. I simply want my mind and body to allow me to live the third part of my life fully; to that end, I do what I can. This does not mean that I don't wish that I had my youthful appearance of my thirties. It just means that I don't go chasing after it. I try to protect my knees and sometimes act in a way that could be interpreted as denial—I exercise too strenuously.

I do spend money on face creams, body lotions, and girl stuff. I hardly own other sorts of cosmetics—in fact, didn't have any until recently, when my daughter stood in front of the cosmetics counter and sweetly said, "Mom, you need some products." I bought some and use them occasionally. She was right: I look better.

Another woman of the same age, a retired college president, wrote this in response to my questions:

When I was young, I thought that people who were in their sixties were really ancient. Now that I am there, I do not feel that way. I suspect like everyone I have a lot of conflicting feelings about getting older. I have found it relatively easy to accept the fact that some of the adventures I hoped to have will not happen (arriving at Machu Picchu by the Inca Trail, climbing Kilimanjaro), but there is plenty left (hiking in the gentler Swiss Alps). I don't have a problem letting people who are younger do things I used to do, like running an impoverished liberal arts college. There are times when I miss the energy that I had, but I still have a lot of energy.

I don't like the memory loss (am I getting Alzheimer's?); and I am most baffled by the uncertainty of how I will age. If I knew, I would be able to make better choices. There is a kind of lack of control over the future that is unsettling to someone who is very used to being in charge. My sister had a stroke when she was sixty-eight—six years older than I. Her mind is fine, but her mobility is limited. A good friend of mine just spent her eighty-second birthday at the Mt. Everest base camp. If I knew which future was closer to mine, I would make the right choices.

I realize that good health is 80 percent of the game. And some people have it, and some don't. Some of it is luck; some of it comes through taking care of oneself. I find myself more patient with older people now and going out of my way to do little things for them. I was less mindful when I was younger.

When I visit my sister in the retirement community, I shudder. And this is when I begin to become afraid and deny. I desperately do not want to be in one of those communities. (I could imagine a rather fun version with about ten friends and lots of space and privacy and luxury.) Every day one is reminded of what is coming, with the Alzheimer's people wandering around and people who can barely move taking half an hour to get down the hall. My denial takes the form of making more commitments to write articles, take on projects, serve on boards—just to say to myself that I'm still young. My inability to deliver may have something to do with age, but more to do with the fact that I do not have a staff of two hundred to pick up the pieces after me. But there is no question that this frenetic pace has something to do with denial.

I desperately want to be able to read books, watch movies, lie in the sun on weekends, but each weekend I am tied to mounds of paper and a computer, and it is catch-up time. Clearly, I am having trouble letting go and accepting a new phase.

Each time I see someone with a botched face-lift, I reaffirm my choice about not having cosmetic surgery. And I do not use makeup.

In the accounts above I note two of the less obvious strategies of denying aging: refusing to give up physical activity that may no longer be appropriate for an older body, and not letting go of patterns of work and mental effort that need to change in order for you to enjoy a slower pace of life in later years. Of course, maintenance of physical and mental activity can also contribute to aging well. It is a question of degree and of the reason for doing it.

The simplest way to deny the fact of growing older is to lie about it. Some people do this so often that they actually do not remember their true age. Do women do this more than men? I don't know. But Oscar Wilde gave this advice: "One should never trust a woman who tells one her real age. A woman who would tell one that would tell one anything."

I see so many middle-aged men who have injured themselves because they did not stop running or playing basketball long after they should have stopped and found other forms of physical activity. I see so many middle-aged women who resort to cosmetic surgery or maintain relentless social and work schedules to keep up with younger women. As I said, denial of aging seems to be the rule in our society, not the exception.

You might wonder how much of it I do. There is nothing like writing a book on aging to force you to confront it in yourself. I do not use antiaging cosmetics and have no interest whatever in cosmetic surgery. I still engage in activities, including some higher-risk ones that might be more appropriate for younger men. (I chased severe storms for a few weeks of the past two summers and got a bit too close to a tornado that tore up the little town of Happy, Texas, on May 5, 2002. This past summer I ran with the bulls during the festival of San Fermín in Pamplona, Spain.) But I assess risks carefully and so far have not come to harm, even if I may have given my guardian angels a lot of work. On the other hand, I have been able to let go of many activities as I have moved away from my youth. In my thirties and forties, I did a great deal of backpacking in wilderness areas. Today, if I consider such trips, I think how nice it would be to have a pack animal rather than carrying all that camping gear on my shoulders.

I like my face as it is and am not in the least tempted to color my beard black, as it was long ago. In fact, looking at my white beard in the mirror gives me good opportunities to reflect on the positive aspects of aging, on the real rewards it can bring.

6

THE VALUE OF AGING

Koko: There is beauty in extreme old age—
Do you fancy you are elderly enough?
Information I'm requesting
On a subject interesting:
Is a maiden all the better when she's tough?

Katisha: Throughout this wide dominion
It's the general opinion
That she'll last a good deal longer when she's tough.

Koko: Are you old enough to marry, do you think?
Won't you wait till you are eighty in the shade?
There's a fascination frantic
In a ruin that's romantic:
Do you think you are sufficiently decayed?

Katisha: To the matter that you mention
I have given some attention.
And I think I am sufficiently decayed.

—Duet of Koko and Katisha from Gilbert and
Sullivan's *The Mikado,* words by
W. S. Gilbert (1885)

I like to ask people to think of examples of things that
improve with age. They never mention maidens these days.

Some common answers are wine, whiskey, cheese, beef, trees, violins, and antiques. I would like to examine the qualities that aging brings out in these things in order to see whether comparable benefits come with aging in people.

Let's begin with drink.

Whiskey and Wine

It is obvious that aged whiskey and wine are more valued than young whiskey and wine, because people are willing to pay a lot more for them. A bottle can cost hundreds or even thousands of dollars. What happens to whiskey and wine in the process of aging that creates such value?

Whiskey—the word comes from a Gaelic term meaning "water of life"—is a distilled liquor made from grain through an intermediate product resembling beer. The grain can be barley, corn, oats, rye, or a mixture of these. All or part of it is first malted—that is, moistened, warmed, and germinated in order to produce enzymes that can convert starch to sugar on which yeast can feed. The yeast is added to a mash of warm water and ground grain, causing a violent, frothing fermentation that eventually quiets down to a liquid called "distiller's beer" with about 8 percent alcohol. This brown liquid is drained from the spent grain and put in a distiller, where it is heated. The vapors, when cooled and condensed, have a much higher alcohol content. Repeated distillations can reduce impurities and raise the alcohol content further. The result is raw whiskey.

What comes out of the distiller is a colorless and mostly flavorless liquid that burns the mouth and throat: firewater. Some raw whiskeys are very high in alcohol—75 percent or more (150 proof or higher). Although some people consume this stuff, mainly as an illegal product ("moonshine," "white lightning," "hooch"), most find it too rough. Such whiskeys are usually diluted with water at a later stage of manufacture. The main reason for aging them in wood is to improve palatability and add flavor, as well as to add color and character.

Whiskey ages only while it is in barrels; once bottled, it undergoes no further change. The alcohol content of the whiskey most of us drink, usually 40 to 50 percent (80 to 100 proof), renders it sterile. A bottle of twelve-year-old Scotch remains a bottle of twelve-year-old Scotch indefinitely.

I am not much of a drinker, but for my money, the best whiskey is single-malt Irish, at least twenty years old. That is not so easy to find, and it is always expensive. A bottle of Bushmills twenty-one-year-old Irish whiskey goes for just under $200.

Aged whiskey is expensive for several reasons. In the first place, some of the product evaporates slowly through the wood. This is known in the trade as the "angels' share"—at least in Ireland, where even angels are thought to participate in the national pastime of consuming alcohol. The result is that the longer the product ages, the less of it there is to bottle. And the angels are thirsty: up to 25 percent of a barrel may be lost to evaporation. Also, a bottle with long-aged contents represents more man-hours and grain acres, not to mention assets that are tied up. But the main reason that whiskey connoisseurs are willing to pay hundreds of dollars for old stuff is that they value its quality. In particular, they talk about mellowness or smoothness as well as depth and complexity of flavor.

To learn more about these positive aspects of aging, I focused on the most famous native American whiskey, Kentucky bourbon. This is made mainly from corn, never less than 51 percent and often 70 percent, with lesser amounts of other grains. It is aged for a minimum of two years, more often four, in new oak barrels that have been charred inside (with a blowtorch or by holding them over a firepot). At the end of aging, the whiskey is filtered through charcoal to remove any particles; contents of several barrels may be blended to produce a consistent product; and water is added to lower the proof to 100 or less. It is then bottled.

As with Irish whiskey and Scotch, really old bourbon is hard to find and costs a lot. Bourbon aficionados say their favorite whiskey is not really drinkable until it has spent twelve years in the barrel and that it comes into its own only after twenty or more years of aging. Consider this description of Old Rip Van Winkle's twelve-year-old Special Reserve, at $40 a bottle: "Luscious, complex toffee and Christmas spice notes. A round, supple entry leads to a dry, expansive medium body. Caramel, nuts, and brown spices are braced by a modest presence of alcohol." Julian Van Winkle III, the third-generation owner of this family distilling business, is one of the pioneers of premium bourbon production. He has said, "My family has always believed that older whiskey has more character and flavor than younger whiskeys. You cannot just age any whiskey and expect it to be good. The whiskey has to be designed to be aged longer." He notes that his bourbon contains a small amount of wheat instead of "cheaper rye," a formula he thinks is better suited for a long time in the barrel.

I called Mr. Van Winkle to ask his thoughts on the positive aspects of aging. "Old whiskey is just more interesting than young, green whiskey," he told me. "It has time to take on all that character of the wood. Of course, you can't just leave a barrel of good bourbon in an overheated upper-story room and expect it to age well. It has to age under the right conditions."

As I said earlier, the aging of whiskey is a chemical process, not a biological one, the result of contact with wood and of limited exposure to air. Some tannins from oak leach into the stored whiskey, giving it more body. Most important, the development of agreeable flavors results directly from contact with the charred inner surface of the oak and with the uncharred wood beneath it.

Wood consists mostly of cellulose and lignins. The latter, which give strength and rigidity to wood, are complicated molecules containing ring structures attached to sugars. When lignins break down under the influence of heat, oxygen, and light, they release aromatic compounds that account for the odors and flavors of familiar spices like nutmeg and cinnamon and, especially, vanilla. The toasting of the insides of oak barrels for both wine and whiskey storage initiates this chemical change. It also causes the caramelization of natural sugars in the wood. These color the whiskey, balance the raw taste of alcohol, and contribute the flavors of caramel and toasted nuts that bourbon drinkers enjoy. The species of oak used is important—some produce much stronger vanilla flavor than others—as is the degree of charring. If it penetrates too deeply into the wood, notes of burn and smoke will overwhelm those of Christmas spices. Finally, evaporation through the barrel concentrates the flavors of the aging whiskey.

To summarize, in the case of whiskey, aging smoothes out rough and raw tastes, adds appealing aromas and flavors, and then concentrates them. In other words, it diminishes undesirable qualities and adds desirable ones, making the product more valuable. Moreover, the processes that develop the desirable qualities, oxidation and caymelization, are the same processes associated with destructive changes in other contexts. Aging cannot make a bad whiskey good, but it can make a good one great. And the environment in which aging occurs—the barrel and how it is stored—is an important determinant of outcome.

Is it necessary to point out the analogies to human aging? We often describe young people as "green" and lacking in depth or complexity of character. Maybe experience cannot make a bad person good, but it can make a good person great. Experience cannot be gained except while undergoing the same processes that cause aspects of aging we think of as destructive, such as sagging of the skin and stiffening of arteries. The benefits and costs of aging cannot be separated. Please remember this truth. If you resist aging, you may deny yourself its benefits. Growing old should increase, not decrease, the value of human life. Just as with bourbon, it has the potential to smooth out roughness, add agreeable qualities, and improve character.

The aging of wine is less understood than the aging of whiskey, because microorganisms play such a great part in the process, even after charred oak barrels have done their work. Wine is a living system in which yeasts, bacteria, and enzymes go on making changes long after the initial fermentation of grape juice. Wine continues to age and often improve in bottles, sometimes over decades. In general, red wines benefit more from aging than whites; they are also more complex. People in many parts of the world enjoy new wines that are light, fruity, uncomplicated, and not intended to last. A prime example is Beaujolais nouveau, released to the world each November within weeks of harvest. But the greatest and most expensive wines in the world are aged.

Château d'Yquem is an extraordinary white wine that, when it has reached maturity, usually at twenty to fifty years, commands prices that are truly astronomical—$480 for a bottle from 1986, $2,200 for a 1921, and $11,550 for an 1878—and sends wine enthusiasts into sensual swoons. It is a sweet dessert wine from the Sauternes district of the Bordeaux region of southwest France, near the Atlantic coast.

This wine has been called "the extravagance of perfection" and has the highest rating *(premier cru classé supérieur)* in the official French system of wine classification. One authority describes it as "intensely opulent when young" and notes that "Yquem develops an extraordinary complexity and exotic richness when fully mature, with the best vintages lasting for over fifty years." The best wines of Château d'Yquem definitely gain in stature as they age, even up to a century if the bottles have been cared for: protected from heat, light, and vibration, and recorked at some point to make sure they remain properly sealed.

I have tasted only a few bottles of Yquem—some younger ones that were wonderful and a twenty-one-year-old that was memorable. I hope sometime to try one that is fifty or older. (I'll let someone else do the buying.) In its youth, this wine is thick and honeylike, with a perfect balance of sweetness and acidity, and a deep, complex flavor. When it ages, all of those qualities are intensified, especially the depth and complexity. Holding a bit of it in your mouth produces an altered state of consciousness.

Production of Yquem is of great interest to me, because it demonstrates a positive potential of decay, a theme I will return to when I write about the aging of cheese. The grapes of Sauternes are susceptible to attack by a mold, *Botrytis cinerea*. Botrytis grows on many fruits and vegetables, usually producing an unappetizing gray rot, but in the environment of Sauternes, it can do something quite magical to grapes. Called *pourriture noble,* or noble rot, it causes them to darken and shrivel and lose water, greatly concentrating the sugar within.

Only fully botrytized grapes are harvested to make the wine of Yquem, and they must be picked one by one over a number of weeks rather than by the bunch all at once. They also have to be handled carefully, because the mold has weakened their skins. This method of harvesting is tedious and time consuming and one reason that Yquem is so costly. Another is that production is small, more so because the volume of juice collected is significantly less than from grapes not affected by noble rot. In fact, yields are so low that each vine produces only one glass of wine.

To make the wine, suitable grapes are quickly pressed, and the juice is fermented in new oak barrels for two or three weeks, sometimes longer, until primary fermentation stops naturally, with the alcohol content about 13.5 percent. The wine then undergoes a long period of barrel aging, during which slow oxidation occurs, as well as secondary fermentation by yeasts and bacteria and an exchange of chemical compounds with the wood. Barrels are topped up twice a week to make up for evaporative loss and racked every three months, meaning that the wine is separated from the lees, or sediment, at the bottom. In the fourth spring after the harvest, wine from different barrels is tasted and blended, and finally bottled. Then it is shipped all over the world, and the mysterious process of aging in the bottle can begin. Here is what Château d'Yquem's Web site has to say about it under the heading "A Hymn to Patience":

> Château d'Yquem has a very long life span: twenty, fifty, a hundred years, or more . . .
>
> As with all great wines, Yquem is transfigured over

time, developing a host of increasingly subtle aromas and flavours. Its colour changes from the brightness of dawn to the darkness of dusk, and from shimmering straw yellow to golden-brown with amber and caramel highlights, and then to translucent mahogany.

Certain connoisseurs consider it outrageous to drink a young Yquem and believe that opening such a monumental wine before its thirtieth birthday is tantamount to a sacrilege.

Aging of wine in the bottle is a combination of enzymatic reactions, slow oxidation, and chemical transformations. You don't need to know the details; even the experts have not worked them out. Suffice it to say that compounds originating in grapes, those created by primary and secondary fermentation, and those coming from wood are broken down with corresponding changes in the color, texture, aroma, and flavor of the wine. With the passage of time, the results are darkening of color, increasing creaminess and thickness of texture, greater complexity of aroma, and greater depth, complexity, and deliciousness of flavor. And, as in the case of whiskey, aging makes wine more valuable.

Cheese

Cheese, in the words of one writer, is "milk's leap toward immortality." It has also been called the "wine of foods"— that is, the food that is closest to wine in its essential nature. Originally invented as a way to preserve milk by concentrating its fat and protein and discarding most of its water, cheese has become a favorite food of many peoples in the Western world, and in some countries (France, Italy, Spain,

Switzerland, and the British Isles especially), the art of cheese making has reached stupendous heights. The key step in the production of the most famous and treasured examples of the cheese maker's art is aging, a process the French call *affinage* and English speakers often call "ripening."

When I listed word associations to the term "old," I discussed ripening in connection with maturity and noted that "ripe" often connotes "rotten" and, therefore, worthless. The word "ripe" is frequently used to describe a cheese in its phase of optimum maturity, but inklings of rottenness are never far from mind, because the most memorable ripe cheeses are often the strong and smelly ones that drive some people wild with anticipation of delight and drive others from the table. Germans have a wonderful collective term for this category of cheeses: *Stinkkäse.*

I have been talking about the concept of aging as the maturing or ripening of a human life. The changes that time brings to whiskey and wine are universally perceived as positive. Who can argue with the value of greater richness, mellowness, and depth of character? But when we consider the breakdown of milk curd by bacteria and molds, the situation is more complex. Some of the odors and flavors that develop are appealing to most Westerners. They remind us of earth, hay, mushrooms, nuts, and other good things. Often, however, especially in the soft-ripened cheeses and most of all in the strong cheeses, these pleasing notes come mixed with hints or overt reminders of decaying vegetation, the barnyard, and even the outhouse.

I will confess here that I am a passionate lover of strong cheeses, very comfortable with the ambivalent sensory experience they provide. Possibly, this is inherited. The family name Weil comes from Alsace, near the area where the borders of France, Germany, and Switzerland meet and home to

Munster, one of the greatest and strongest cheeses in the world (and no relation to the bland cheese of the same name that Americans buy in supermarkets). When I was growing up, my father's mother lived with us at various times, and she and my father introduced me at an early age to the joy of eating fragrant cheese, much to the horror of my mother, whose family came from the Ukraine and who had to leave the table when we indulged. Our favorite was Liederkranz, once available in the refrigerated dairy sections of most supermarkets, and, to my taste, the greatest cheese that America has ever produced. Sadly, it is no longer made.

If you thought whiskey making and wine making were complicated, I can only tell you that they pale into simplicity beside the making of fine cheese. So many things can go wrong. In particular, the wrong organisms can grow and dominate the cheese, not only ones that create bitterness and other off flavors but some that can reduce it to a slimy mess.

I was planning a trip to Alsace to learn about the manufacture of real cheese and eat my fill of ripe Munster, when I discovered a source of information much closer to home. I read an article in *The New Yorker* about Sister Noella Marcellino, a cloistered nun at the Benedictine Abbey of Regina Laudis in Bethlehem, Connecticut, who makes very traditional, very living cheese and has become an internationally renowned expert on the subject. I wrote Sister Noella of my interest, but it took some time to get a response, because she was preparing to defend her thesis, the last hurdle she had to clear to obtain her doctorate in microbiology from the University of Connecticut. (The title of the thesis, which I later read, is "The Biodiversity of *Geotrichum candidum* Strains Isolated from Traditional French Cheese.") When she learned of my intent to draw lessons from the aging of cheese that might apply to human aging, she immediately understood, saw the relevance of teachings in her own spiritual tradition, and invited me to the abbey.

I spent a few wonderful days there in the fall of 2003. The Abbey of Regina Laudis is a unique institution that is home to thirty-nine nuns, many of whom were successful in the world as lawyers, scholars, artists, and corporate executives before they took their vows. The foundress of the abbey, Right Reverend Mother Benedict Duss, encourages them to continue their art and scholarship within the order. It was she who sent Sister Noella back to school to get a higher degree in her chosen branch of agricultural science.

Sister Noella—she is now officially Mother Noella, having taken her final vows—turned out to be a beaming, delightful companion as well as a good teacher and a fount of information about cheese and cheese making. She is irrepressible in spirit, humor, and energy. I am tempted to add "uncloisterable," because of her very visible presence in the world. She is now the subject of a video documentary, "The Cheese Nun: Sister Noella's Voyage of Discovery," and shortly after our visit she traveled to Paris to be honored by the French government for her work in promoting awareness of natural cheeses and the traditional art of making them. But she is very much part of the remarkable life of a fully cloistered, religious community.

I won't burden you with the technical details of the chemistry of cheese making and cheese ripening. I will just say that the same processes of decay and putrefaction responsible for the rotting of organic matter can, in controlled circumstances, result in living foods of great nutritional value and appeal. Unaged Camembert, Brie, and Munster are green, one-dimensional, and uninteresting. With age, they develop the colors, textures, and flavors that make them great.

I had a long conversation about aging with Sister Noella. She focused immediately on the positive aspects of decay and putrefaction. In the hands of a skilled cheese maker they create perfection, she said. She also talked about the range of odors and flavors associated with cheese that can be unpleasant. We discussed frankly the desirability of embracing both the attractive and repellent aspects of life—not only in eating cheese but in accepting the inevitable decay of our bodies.

That night, as I lay in bed in the men's guesthouse, after lots of cheese and homemade bread, I turned over in my mind the idea of aging as ripening. We do not think of ripe fruit as having aged to reach ripeness, but it certainly has endured, allowing time to soften its texture, change its starches to sugars, and create appetizing colors and flavors, all intended to entice us and other animals to eat it and so disperse the seeds within. Of course, the ripening of fruit is a metabolic process that does not involve the chemistry of putrefaction, so we are not ambivalent about it. Nonetheless, the stage of perfect ripeness of fruit precedes a decline into overripeness and decay, just as with cheese.

When I look at other aspects of nature, I see a similar sequence. A glorious sunset at the end of day is the ripening of the daily cycle, just before the plunge into night. The magnificence of autumn foliage is the ripe period of the year, before the sleep of winter. Yes, our bodies will decline and decay, but aging, if accepted and not resisted, can lead to maturity and all of the promise implied in the colors of sunset and fall foliage, in the perfection of ripe fruit and the pleasure of expertly aged cheese.

I still have some Bethlehem cheese in my refrigerator, and when I taste it, all the memories of the Abbey of Regina Laudis come back in full vividness. Sister Noella writes that she is very busy and spending much of her time in choir. "Do you think singing helps with healthy aging?" she asks. "I do."

Beef

"Beef, like fine wine, improves with age." So says the Beef Information Centre, a division of the Canadian Cattlemen's Association, and steak lovers agree. They are willing to pay premium prices for properly aged, high-grade cuts of beef, because aging produces two desirable changes in their favorite meat: it makes it more tender and increases its flavor.

Tenderness of meat has to do with the cut (how much connective tissue it has), the grade (how much fat is marbled in the muscle tissue), the method of cooking, and whether or not it is aged. Many factors also go into the determination of flavor, one of them being concentration as a result of water loss during the traditional method of aging. That is dry aging, in which a whole carcass is hung, uncovered, in a refrigerated room with circulating air and constant, moderate humidity—not the newer, quicker, cheaper, and much inferior method that has largely replaced it.

I have not eaten meat in more than thirty years, being a pesco-lacto-vegetarian. That is, I live mostly on fish and vegetables, and except for cheese (and very occasional eggs) I do not eat other animal products. How, then, am I qualified to discuss the virtues of aged beef? Well, before I gave up meat I ate my share of steak, and I always wondered why steak in good restaurants tasted so much better than steak cooked at home. My father, who was a meat-and-potatoes man, explained that aging was responsible. His father had been a butcher in Philadelphia, and he described to me the cold lockers in which sides of beef were hung for weeks, often becoming covered with thick layers of mold. He pointed out that the fat of aged beef is cream-colored rather than white, that its texture is buttery, and its flavor is intense.

These changes result not from microbial action—the surface mold is incidental and must be scraped off—but from enzymatic processes that occur in muscle tissue after death. "Postmortem aging" is the technical term, but "ripening" is also sometimes used. "Still no one denies that dry aging is basically controlled rotting," writes the owner of one top steakhouse. That sounds familiar.

Shortly after an animal is slaughtered, its muscles go into rigor mortis, a condition of rigidity that lasts from a few hours to a day. As you can imagine, it is during this time that meat will be least tender. Once rigor mortis ends and dead muscles relax, they begin to break down under the influence of protein-digesting enzymes in cells. This process, called proteolysis, releases flavorful amino acids that are the constituents of less flavorful proteins. The enzymes also soften the connective tissue that accounts for some of the toughness of meat.

Meat aging today is done at temperatures just above freezing, with just the right amounts of humidity and air circulation to minimize the growth of spoilage-causing bacteria. Still, there is much disagreement over how long beef should be kept in these conditions to achieve optimum flavor and tenderness. My former college roommate, the well-known food writer Jeffrey Steingarten, has this to say on the subject:

> Research shows that the maximum increase in tenderness is achieved at three weeks of dry aging. But the fla-

vor keeps developing from the initial fresh, iron-meaty taste to a round, buttery, complex, and mouthwatering savor. Eight weeks seems just right to me.

Again, aging intensifies the desirable characteristics of a food through concentration of flavor and transformation of less desirable qualities into more desirable ones. You just have to start with good raw materials, provide the right conditions, and be patient.

Trees

I once slogged uphill for hours through deep mud and driving rain in a faraway place just to see a tree. Of course, it was not an ordinary tree. It was one of the most remarkable trees of the world, an ancient sugi *(Cryptomeria japonica)* on Yakushima, a circular island due south of Kyushu, the southernmost of Japan's main islands.

Sugis are often called cedars, but they are not related to true cedars. The particular one I was climbing to see, called the Jomon Cedar, is said to be 7,200 years old and a relic of the Jomon era, the earliest period in Japanese history. That is unlikely. There is as much local incentive to exaggerate the ages of old trees as of old people. The Jomon Cedar (or Jomon Sugi), though, may be over 2,000 years old and is certainly the largest conifer in Japan, possibly bigger than any in Europe. When I got to it, deep within the dripping forest, it was more than worth the muddy climb—a gnarled giant that is the closest thing I have seen in the real world to an Ent, one of the mythical tree beings that help the heroes of J. R. R. Tolkien's *Lord of the Rings*. I sat at its feet, half expecting to hear it speak in a deep, woody voice. I wanted to stay in its presence, but I soon got too soaked and had to say good-bye.

There are a number of huge, old sugi trees on Yakushima, a major reason that the forests of that island have been designated a World Heritage Property and put under strict protection. We value old trees. I seek them out, whether they are famous or not.

Let me tell you about a few other famous ones I know. I have visited the venerable Tule Tree of southern Mexico several times. It is a Montezuma cypress *(Taxodium mucronatum)*, and it grows in a little town east of the city of Oaxaca, next to the Church of Santa Maria del Tule, which it dwarfs with its magnificent bulk. Its massive trunk—it has the largest girth of any tree in the world—is mostly covered by a dense canopy of feathery leaves.

Members of the genus *Taxodium*, which are related to coast redwoods and giant sequoias, can grow very fast if they have abundant water. "Tule" means "marsh" in the local Zapotec dialect, and this particular *Taxodium* got going in a reedy marsh fed by two rivers well over 2,000 years ago. But in 1994, it began to die. Experts diagnosed the problem as lack of water. The marsh had been drained, the rivers diverted, a town built on the site. Panic struck the nation and the state of Oaxaca, forcing governments to take action. They rerouted traffic and brought water to the tree. It recovered.

I have also spent time camping beneath the biggest trees in the world, the giant sequoias *(Sequoiadendron giganteum)* in the Sierra Nevada mountains of central California, some of which may have been growing for 700 or 800 years, I have seen huge old camphor trees *(Cinnamomum camphora)* on the grounds of shrines in Japan, including one in the seaside resort town of Atami that is considered especially sacred. Shinto priests decorate it with ropes and paper tassels, and the faithful make pilgrimages in order to circumambulate it: each circuit is supposed to add a year to your life. I have tipped my hat to old, hollow baobabs *(Adansonia digitata)* in Africa, their swollen trunks looking as if they had been inflated with air pumps. I have sat reverently beneath enormous copper beeches on Long Island and craned my neck to look up into the massive branches of some of the few old-growth Douglas firs *(Pseudotsuga menziesii)* remaining in the Pacific Northwest.

To me, it is the great age of all these trees that makes them special, not their size. Very old trees have a presence about them, a gravity, that draws you in, makes you quiet, and fills you with awe and respect. Sit in front of some old bonsai trees and note how you feel. Bonsai—the Japanese word means "tray planting"*—is the ancient art of dwarfing trees by cultivating them in small, shallow containers. Bonsai originated in China but developed into a distinctive art form in Japan. You can view old bonsai trees with great presence in the arboretums and botanical gardens of major cities, both here and in the Far East. The National Arboretum in Washington, D.C., has a fine collection, as do the Arnold Arboretum in Boston and the Brooklyn Botanic Garden. Many specimens are over a hundred years old, some two hundred, a few four hundred. An adult human can dwarf one of these dwarfed trees, but I submit that their gravity and presence are every bit as powerful as those of the gigantic trees I have mentioned above.

There are several methods of creating exact replicas in living miniature of great, old trees. One is to search for trees

---

*Pronounced *bone-sigh* and not to be confused with *banzai*, the Japanese victory shout meaning "ten thousand years."

in the wild that are naturally stunted as a result of growing in hostile circumstances. For example, in the desert Southwest, where I live, you could look in the upper reaches of canyons for junipers lodged in crevices of rocks, with minimal soil and water. If you find one with just the right size and form, you could try carefully digging it out of the rock, transplanting it to a pot, and then, if it survives the move, you could gradually trim its roots and accustom it to living in a tray. Japanese bonsai artists are sometimes accused of cruelty to plants, but, actually, ancient bonsai are revered as cultural treasures, are pampered, and generally live longer than most of their counterparts in the wild.

The oldest trees in the world are not massive but naturally stunted. The bristlecone pines *(Pinus longaeva)* that grow high up (10,000 feet above sea level) in the White Mountains on the California-Nevada border and in a few other inhospitable locations, look as if they are barely alive. These small, gnarled trees with many snags and dead branches grow on rocky ledges in sites with little water, extremes of temperature, high winds, and strong solar radiation. Some are over 4,000 years old. Doubtless, it is the very hostility of the environment that forces them to slow their life processes to a minimum and grow very slowly.

Biogerontologists like to disparage claims of longevity made for old trees. Here is Leonard Hayflick on the subject:

Annual growth rings are counted in woody trees to determine a tree's chronological age, but the cells in nearly all of those rings are dead. Just beneath the outermost ring of dead bark in a woody tree lies the living cambium layer. Further inside, one finds more dead cells. Thus, the band of living cells is sandwiched between the dead bark and the dead internal annual rings. By weight or by volume most of the substance of the trunk of an old tree is composed of dead cells. . . . Most of the oldest bristlecone pines cling to life by a narrow ribbon of living tissue that snakes up the wall of the dead trunk. The oldest *living* cells in a redwood tree, giant sequoia, or bristlecone pine can be found in the needles and the cones, and they are no more than twenty or thirty years of age. That is why, if you are past your thirtieth birthday, I insist that you are older than what some mistakenly call the world's "oldest" trees!

I think this is beside the point. We have no trouble distinguishing a living tree from a dead one. The ancient bristlecone pines may be barely alive, but they still grow new needles when environmental conditions are right, and they still produce cones with viable seeds and so pass on their life to their progeny. The point is that these organisms have survived, not what percentage of them is composed of living cells. Very old trees have survived storms, floods, lightning strikes, earthquakes, forest fires, diseases, predators, and, perhaps most of all, the saws and axes of loggers. Bigger, older trees often provide more valuable timber; as logging makes them scarce, their worth increases, as does the incentive to harvest them. Old trees, like old whiskey and wine, certainly have more character than young trees, but that is not the main reason that we venerate them, consider them sacred, and make pilgrimages to see them. We honor them because they are survivors.

Moreover, their appearance is often testimony to their past struggles. Many of the oldest trees are not conventionally beautiful. They are scarred, ragged, twisted, and gnarled, and we love them for it, because their imperfections only reinforce the fact of their endurance. No one would want to see these Methuselahs of the woods undergo cosmetic surgery or receive some sort of Botox-for-trees to make them smoother and straighter. Any such treatment would lessen their gravity and its effect on visitors.

Written in the shapes and forms of old trees are experience and wisdom—experience of many seasons and many changes, wisdom of how to adapt to those changes. Is it special genetics that allows a very few individual trees to attain great longevity? Is it just luck and circumstance?

When I see old people who are proud of their aging and not ashamed of it, I see in them the same kind of wisdom and experience. Old people are survivors who have avoided the pitfalls of reckless youth and the common failings of middle age. I do not regard their white hair and wrinkled faces as signs of frailty or detractions from human beauty. I see those features as the banners of survivorship.

Violins

It is common knowledge that some old violins are priceless, costing millions of dollars if they ever come on the market, and that some of the greatest violinists in the world own and play such instruments. The best known are those produced by Antonio Stradivari (1644?–1737) and the Guarneri family, especially Giuseppe Guarneri (1687–1745). They are magnificent instruments—and they have improved with age. And, as with whiskey and wine, the better the violin to begin with, the better it becomes with age.

At the end of the nineteenth century, well before the advent of the phonograph and radio, violins were in great demand for live entertainment. A great many cheap, mass-market instruments were produced at that time in eastern Germany and adjacent Bohemia, now part of the Czech Republic. If you look through American mail-order catalogs of the period, you will find these violins advertised, with price tags ranging from two to fifty dollars. And if you find any of them today, whether they are 100 or 150 years old, they will not have gained much in value. The reasons? They were cheaply made to begin with, and there are so many of them.

"But if a violin is well made, time will improve it," says Richard Ward, an expert with Ifshin Violins in Berkeley, California, a company that makes violins and restores and appraises old ones. "Violins have to mature. Even those of the great masters took forty to eighty years to come into their own. Many skilled makers of violins today are producing fine instruments that sell for high prices. But they sound *new*. They need time and playing to mature."

I soon discovered that no one understands this process, because, again, there are too many variables. "It may have to do with oxidation of the varnish," Ward speculates. (And we know that oxidation is a change common to the aging of many things, including us.) "It may have to do with the drying of wood over time or with its experience of repeated vibration. Some kinds of instruments age differently from others, but most good violins need at least fifty years of playing to mature and produce the optimum sound they are capable of. Even after that, they may continue to improve with aging."

But Ward also pointed out another interesting fact about these instruments: "If an old violin surfaces—a good one—that has been well cared for but hasn't been played in fifty years, it may again sound new. It will have to be played, over time, to get back its former capacity."

I see in this story benefits of aging I have already noted—in particular, the augmentation of desirable qualities by changes that time brings, changes that in other contexts might appear destructive. In addition, there is the phenomenon of maturing through experience, perhaps unexpected in an inanimate object. And there is another aspect of value here, one that I will comment on in the following section: old violins are connections to the past, direct links to the genius and secrets of the master violin makers of three centuries ago.

Antiques

It has been popular over the years to make fun of collectors of antiques and their willingness to pay good money for what some people consider old junk. That attitude has diminished recently, because of wide publicity given to stories of collectors striking it rich—for example, on the popular *Antiques Roadshow* on American public television. The *Roadshow* travels around the country, bringing experts together with collectors and ordinary folks who trot out items from their attics and basements to have them identified and appraised. Of course, many of those items are worth little, even if they are old and the owners are fond of them. But, not infrequently, lucky people learn that their possessions are worth fortunes.

A Tucson couple named Ted and Virginia brought a Navajo blanket to *Roadshow* appraiser Donald Ellis in 2002. Ted said the blanket had been in his family for years; his grandmother used to put it on the foot of his bed when he was a boy in case he got cold during the night. "We weren't particularly in love with it," he said. "It was nice, but it wasn't particularly colorful like our Navajo rugs. We just threw it over the back of a rocking chair in the bedroom, and nothing was ever said about it. We thought it might be worth two, three, or four thousand dollars." But Ellis recognized it as an early example of an unusual style of Navajo blanket, dating from about 1840 and in remarkably good condition: no holes, no fading, with an exceptionally tight weave and silky-smooth finish. He appraised it at almost half a million dollars, and it sold for that amount at the New York City Winter Antiques Show in January 2003.

Why is an old, not particularly colorful blanket worth so much money? Why are some antiques so valuable, often in spite of their lack of intrinsic beauty or appeal? One answer is that they are rare. In the mid-1800s, many Navajo blankets of this type were probably in circulation, and their prices reflected the actual costs of materials, labor, quality, and distribution. But over the years that style and quality of weaving became uncommon, and one after another of the blankets disappeared. Some were lost, some destroyed by moths or fire, some faded by exposure to sunlight, until few remained, and of those, even fewer were near perfect. With the passage of time, they become ever rarer and consequently ever more valuable.

Another reason is that such a blanket, like a Stradivarius violin in good condition, is a tangible link to the past. It was made, handled, and used by Native Americans who lived two decades before the American Civil War, when Navajos were part of a West as yet unsettled and unpacified. Sleep under it or throw it over a rocking chair if you like, but, most likely, it will become part of a museum or private collection, a focus of attention and admiration as a surviving remnant of a distant time. The older the object, the greater its power to fascinate. I have twice been to the Egyptian

Museum in Cairo to view antiquities and have twice leaned over the glass case containing the mummy of Rameses II, my face inches from his. This was the Pharaoh who ruled during the time of the Exodus. How incredible that any relic of him survives into our time! I want to look on that face again.

Obviously, we fuss so much over centenarians because they are rare. The percentage of people who survive at least into their nineties is low, even lower for those who do so in good condition. As I told you earlier, traditional Okinawans regard their oldest citizens as living treasures and make great efforts to include them in all community activities. Our culture could benefit from adopting a similar attitude.

A common sentiment I hear in connection with antiques is, If only they could speak, what stories they could tell. Old people can speak and tell their stories. When aging parents and grandparents are part of extended families and not isolated in institutions, they serve as links to the past for children and young adults. I remember as a child listening to my grandmother's stories of the Blizzard of '88. That was 1888, when she was a little girl in Philadelphia. The storm, said to be the most famous snowstorm in American history, paralyzed the Northeast in mid-March, high winds and snow creating drifts forty and fifty feet high. I would know nothing of it and certainly feel none of its immediacy except for her account. I also remember both her and my mother describing the influenza pandemic of 1918 in Philadelphia. I was riveted by my grandmother's descriptions of horse-drawn carts carrying corpses of flu victims through the streets. It sounded like a scene from the Middle Ages in Europe, not something that could have happened in Philadelphia in the living memory of someone in my family.

At the time I heard their stories—in the early 1950s— memory of the flu pandemic of 1918 was strongly repressed in our society. Only recently has it surfaced, finally become the subject of books and video documentaries, and stimulated scientific investigation. Infectious-disease experts now recognize the urgency of finding out why the virus of 1918 was so virulent, why it was able to kill healthy, young adults so quickly. They know we are due for another pandemic and want us to be prepared. I've been thinking about all this since the 1950s, because an older person in my life connected me to that momentous and tragic time. Old people are our links to our history. As you age, your worth in this respect increases.

My intention in this discussion has been to direct your thinking toward areas of human experience where the value of aging is obvious. I have used these examples to show that aging has the potential to bring greater worth to human life. It can:

- add richness to life
- replace the shallowness and greenness of youth with depth and maturity
- develop and enhance desirable qualities of personality while lessening undesirable ones
- smooth out roughness of character
- enhance the mental, emotional, and spiritual aspects of life by the same processes that cause decline of the physical body
- confer the advantages and power of survivorship
- develop one's voice and authority as a living link to the past.

I want to conclude this chapter with a few additional thoughts and questions. Remember that what gives value to the things I have described is not what is on the outside but what is within. And remember the importance of patience: you must resist the urge to try fine wine or cheese prematurely. From where I am now, I cannot imagine what I will be at eighty, any more than I can envision a sapling becoming a great, old tree. What are the optimal conditions for human aging to produce greatness? What part of ourselves needs to evaporate in order to concentrate our essence? What do we have to let go?

My main hope for this book is that it will, in whatever measure possible, begin to change the harmful conception most people have of aging: that it diminishes the worth of living. I am under no illusions about the difficulty of this task. Unrelenting images and messages come at us from the media telling us that youth is where it's at, that growing old is a disaster, that the worth of life peaks early. I can only tell you as clearly and strongly as I can that I disagree, and I ask you to look to the examples above and to other areas of your experience to discover and realize the value of aging.

7

INTERLUDE: JENNY

Shortly after I wrote the last chapter, my mother died. She was ninety-three, and although her death was expected— she had been declining for the past year—it nonetheless came as a shock to her many friends. Jenny Weil had so much energy for most of her life and was so sharp mentally that many people thought she would go on forever. She didn't, but she remains for me and many others a model of graceful aging.

My mother loved to travel and went all over the world with my father. After he died in 1993, I took her with me on trips to Canada, Japan, and Europe. This was by no means a chore. She was a lot of fun to travel with and made friends wherever she went.

When Jenny was eighty-eight, she slipped on a tiled floor, fell, and broke her pelvis. The fracture healed quickly but left her, for the first time, fearful about venturing out on her own. I thought a successful trip might get her over this and offered to take her anywhere she wanted to go for her eighty-ninth birthday that January. She announced that she wanted to go to Antarctica. So we went—not the easiest trip for someone her age, but she did fine and came back with renewed confidence and vitality. The next summer, she accompanied me, my daughter, and friends on a week of whale watching in a small boat in southeast Alaska. We saw many humpback whales at close range, but Jenny wanted to get even closer to them. The naturalist in charge offered to take her and me out in a motorized raft. Soon after we got away from the boat, a huge whale came up very near our little raft, a thrilling encounter for me. But when Jenny got back to the boat, where our friends had watched it all through binoculars, she said, "Not close enough."

A year later, she went with a much younger woman on a trip to New York to stay with a friend of mine. Here is that friend's report of their first day:

> Jenny and Suzi arrived at my apartment after one of those nightmare trips into the city from the airport. Jenny wanted to hit the pavement right away. We had tickets for the theater that night, but she insisted on first going to the Met [the Metropolitan Museum of Art]. We walked from my apartment at 90th [Street] and Central Park West to 72nd [Street] and Third Avenue, where there was a street fair. Jenny walked up and down the Avenue seeking out hat stands. [She and my father had owned a millinery supply shop in Philadelphia for many years.] She was enthralled with the hats and delighted in showing us which were the best ones. Then we went to the Met and did the Impressionists, then out to dinner and the theater, and finally got back to my apartment, where Suzi and I were ready to collapse. Jenny said, "That was a really nice day, but I wish we could have done more."

Jenny was then ninety. I took great pleasure in showing her off. She was charming, elegant, and witty. She remembered in great detail her last meeting with someone, even if that person had forgotten it. She always asked how *you* were, what *you* were doing, before she talked about herself. She had a fine sense of humor, liked to point out the ridiculous side of life, and was able to get many people to laugh with her. She had a large circle of true friends, people from all over the world she had made strong connections with, people of all ages, of many cultures, of very different social backgrounds.

Jenny didn't like it when I told people her age, and she didn't want to slow down. One day she came to my home for dinner when I was entertaining a doctor and his wife from India. The doctor headed an Ayurvedic spa in Mysore that I had visited. He invited Jenny to come there, enticing her with descriptions of various rejuvenating therapies she could have. She listened politely, then said firmly, "I don't want to be rejuvenated."

She did want to go to India, though, and Tibet—two places she hadn't been. And she was determined to ride the full length of the Trans-Siberian Railroad with a young, adventurous friend. This was not to be.

At age ninety-one, Jenny began slowing down. She complained about not having enough "pep," about running out of energy. I noticed mild cognitive impairment, mainly difficulty in remembering names, though nothing that seemed abnormal for her age. Occasionally, I heard her say that being old was no fun, but that was very rare. Then, while visiting me in British Columbia in 2003, she had an episode of acute heart failure, which manifested itself as sudden shortness of breath. In the hospital, she was found to have severe aortic stenosis, extreme narrowing of the heart valve that admits oxygen-rich blood to the main artery supplying the whole body. Jenny's body and brain had been subsisting on minimal nourishment. We had never known her to have a heart problem. This was clearly an age-related disease. Her aortic valve had become calcified and stiff after so many years of constant work.

There is a surgical treatment for aortic stenosis: replacement of the worn-out valve with a good one from a pig, but my mother was adamant about not wanting to undergo surgery, and her cardiologist and I agreed it would not be a wise course. There was too great a risk that Jenny would come out of the operation with a better-functioning heart but an impaired brain. So we decided to treat her medically, with drugs to keep fluid from accumulating in her lungs and to help her heart pump more efficiently. The prognosis was not good: a high chance of worsening heart failure and a high risk of sudden cardiac death.

Jenny responded to the medication, but her life was not the same. Walking became difficult for her, partly from shortness of breath and partly from a knee injury resulting from another fall a few months earlier. Her concentration was impaired, probably from diminished blood flow to the brain, making it hard for her to read or even watch videos. She became alarmingly thin, despite everyone's best efforts to encourage her to eat. Getting her out of her apartment to a restaurant, a movie, or anywhere became more and more of a chore, yet she kept talking about trips to Tibet and Siberia.

Jenny's doctor, a cardiologist who is an old, good friend of mine, says she became his favorite patient because of her spunk and optimism. "She never failed to ask me about my wife and kids, whom she knew well," he recalls, "and she always said she was getting better. She always made me laugh."

Jenny went into and out of heart failure over her last

year and was mostly confined to her apartment in her last few months. She did not have to move to an assisted-living facility, stayed out of the hospital, and died suddenly at home, after a full day of interacting with visitors and receiving many calls from friends and family. Her exit was private, dignified, and blessedly quick.

My mother lived much longer than her parents and most of her siblings. She enjoyed good health almost all of her life, arrived in her nineties with most of her faculties intact, and had a relatively quick decline in her last year, with minimal medical intervention—the compression of morbidity that we all should seek. Certainly, her body aged. In going through old photographs from her album in preparation for a memorial celebration of her life, I was astonished at the degree of physical change over the years, from a beautiful newlywed to a somewhat heavyset young mother to a trim and fit older woman and finally to the wise elder she became. But I think it is fair to say that *she* did not age, even if her body did. She was verbally deft, mentally sharp, and witty to the day of her death and had acquired real wisdom in the course of her long life, wisdom that she shared.

My mother had a great deal of practical knowledge and skill—about plants, about domestic matters, about life—and people sought her out for advice on many subjects. She was a masterful seamstress and mender as a result of her long experience in making ladies' hats. She could remove any sort of stain from any sort of fabric, a talent I have not inherited. And she had a very consistent philosophy that enabled her to ride out the ups and downs of life with equanimity. Her motto, often repeated, was: "No matter what happens to you in life, never lose your sense of humor."

I have come to realize that Jenny's last and lasting gift to me was the timing of her death—just as I was about to turn from writing about the science and philosophy of aging to the practicalities of it. I want to know what she did right that enabled her to avoid the cancers that killed her mother and two of her sisters prematurely and the Alzheimer's disease that engulfed her father. What got her through the experience of a fractured pelvis at age eighty-nine so quickly that she was off to Antarctica a few months later? How was it that she still had her wits about her, still came across as witty and wise, and was still able to make people laugh even on the last day of her life, when her brain had been getting a fraction of the blood it needed and her heart was no longer capable of working against such mechanical resistance? These questions fascinate me. I believe they have answers, answers that are consistent with the practical information I am about to give you in the second part of this book.

PART TWO

How to Age Gracefully

8

BODY I: THE OUNCE
OF PREVENTION

In the following chapters, I will give you my recommendations for what you can do to increase the probability of
experiencing healthy aging. These prescriptions follow from
the scientific and philosophical considerations in the first
part of this book. Therefore, they are not intended to help
you grow younger, to extend life beyond its reasonable limits, or to make it easier for you to deny the fact of aging. The
goal is to adapt to the changes that time brings and to arrive
in old age with minimal deficits and discomforts—in technical terms, to compress morbidity. You want to be able to
savor life even in its latter years and to manifest, enjoy, and
share with others the genuine rewards that aging can
bestow.

I have organized this part of the book into sections con-
cerning body, mind, and spirit. I will begin by discussing the
needs of the physical body, focusing particularly on diet,
activity, and rest. In the section on mind, I include recommendations about stress, thoughts, and emotions and their
influences on health and aging, as well as tips for avoiding
age-related deficits of memory. Finally, I will ask you to consider that aspect of yourself that is not physical and does not
change through time: spirit. I believe that healthy aging

depends in part on awareness of one's spiritual identity and discovery of ways to enhance the interactions of spirit with body and mind.

Your body has grown and developed according to the genetic instructions acquired from your parents and contained within every cell. As scientists continue to identify the products and functions of our genes—the sequencing of the human genome is one of the greatest achievements of our time—they are demonstrating the far-reaching influence of genetics on all aspects of life, including aging. They are also creating possibilities for new kinds of medical interventions that may blunt the expression of diseases and optimize human potentials. Studies of monozygotic (identical) twins consistently emphasize the importance of genetics in determining not only most of the physical characteristics of the body but also many of our intellectual, emotional, and behavioral traits. At the same time, research also consistently reminds us of the profound influence of environment on genes and their expression. It is always nature *and* nurture, never just one or the other. Nature has dealt you a certain hand of genetic cards, some good, some not so good; it is up to you how to play them.

As an example, consider the many factors that affect a woman's risk of developing breast cancer over her lifetime. Clearly, there is a genetic component of risk, not only as a result of specific, known genes that greatly increase the possibility of early-onset (before age fifty) breast cancer, but also in familial patterns that make the disease more likely if more female blood relatives (mothers, sisters, aunts) are affected. Yet, if we look at all cases of breast cancer, only a minority of them can properly be called inherited. Most result from increased stimulation of breast cells by estrogen, from failures of immune defenses, and from exposure to known toxins.

Women differ in how much estrogen they produce, in how they metabolize it, and in how many years of their lives their breast tissue is exposed to high levels of it. There are genetic influences here along with environmental ones. Early onset of menstruation and late onset of menopause both increase lifetime estrogen exposure, while having babies and breast-feeding both decrease it. The body metabolizes estrogen along two main enzymatic pathways. One leads to a metabolite that increases breast cancer risk, the other does not; it may even reduce risk. A woman's genes may influence the preferred pathway, but so do her dietary habits. Cruciferous (cabbage-family) vegetables contain a compound (I-3-C) that shifts estrogen metabolism into the pathway of reduced risk. Women concerned about breast cancer because of their family histories can eat these vegetables regularly or take the isolated compound as a dietary supplement. On the other hand, alcohol, even in moderation, can shift estrogen metabolism to the more dangerous route. The risk of breast cancer is increased among women who prefer meat well done. The hotter and longer animal tissue is cooked, the higher its content of carcinogenic toxins.

The message here is that environmental factors, including many that you control, influence the final expression of genes. My mother did not develop the diseases that shortened the lives of her parents and sisters. Maybe she had different inherited risks. Certainly, she was more knowledgeable than they were about lifestyle and health, and she was both able and determined to take better care of herself as she advanced in age. You can do the same.

Taking care of the body means different things at different stages in life. For example, accidents are major causes of death and disability in people in their teens and twenties, many the results of thoughtless or reckless behavior, such as riding motorcycles without helmets, diving headfirst into murky bodies of water, and using drugs and alcohol unwisely. Habits acquired in these years—notably addiction to tobacco—can markedly increase the risk of chronic disease in later life. Men in their thirties and forties often injure themselves as a result of engaging in contact sports or exercising improperly, while men in their fifties and sixties are often too sedentary. One of the secrets of healthy aging is knowing how to evaluate the riskiness of your behavior. Another is willingness to let go of behaviors more suited to younger bodies.

You will not have a chance to experience healthy aging if you fall into one of the common pitfalls that claim people in midlife, such as a heart attack or a tobacco-related cancer. To avoid these, you must be aware of your personal health risks as suggested by your past medical history, your family history, and medical examinations. You also need to know how to take advantage of modern preventive medicine—for example, how to make the best use of diagnostic screening tests now available.

This last subject is not so simple. Just because a test is available does not mean you should take it. Tests may not be accurate or sensitive enough to justify their use. They may indicate problems where none exist (false positives) or miss existing ones (false negatives). If they indicate disease for which no treatment is available or for which available treatments are inadequate and potentially dangerous, the benefit to you may be minimal. Consider a few examples.

Screening for hypertension—high blood pressure—is now routine. Measurement of blood pressure is fast, simple, and noninvasive. Treatment for hypertension is also good. Many cases can be normalized with low doses of medications that are relatively safe and relatively free of side effects, such as beta-blockers and diuretics. Control of hypertension is one of the great medical advances of the second half of the twentieth century and is doubtless one of the factors responsible for the declining rate of heart attacks in this period. Elevated blood pressure damages the entire cardiovascular system over time and can impair kidney function—major causes of age-related diseases and avoidable pitfalls.

In our society, and in developed countries generally, blood pressure increases with age, perhaps because of our dietary habits, the stress of modern life, and other unknown factors. (It does not do so in "primitive" tribal cultures.) The start of this process can often be detected early in life, and doctors are increasingly eager to diagnose it and treat it. Not long ago, many cases were dismissed as "borderline" hypertension or "labile" hypertension that varied wildly from reading to reading. Now the trend is to call all of this "prehypertension" and to treat it aggressively. I prefer that people with this label monitor their own blood pressure at home for a month or two to get a better picture of it (automatic cuffs with digital readouts are inexpensive and very easy to use) and first try lifestyle measures to normalize it: losing weight, increasing exercise, practicing relaxation techniques, taking dietary supplements (magnesium, for example), eating fewer foods high in sodium and more vegetables. But if the trend is still toward hypertension after a reasonable trial period, say, eight weeks, then I recommend antihypertensive medication, starting with the lowest dose of the mildest drug.

Cholesterol screening is not as clear cut, in my opinion. You should definitely know your levels of total cholesterol,

HDL and LDL, and serum triglycerides (along with serum homocysteine, an independent risk factor for heart attack, and C-reactive protein, an indicator of inflammation in arteries). Most doctors now favor treatment with statin drugs if these values are abnormal; some cardiologists say they would like to see statins added to the water supply. I am not quite that sanguine about them for several reasons. In the first place, statins are not as benign as the first-level antihypertensive drugs. Statins can disturb liver and muscle function, sometimes seriously. Second, coronary heart disease is multifactorial, involving abnormal inflammation, many influences of heredity and lifestyle, and a significant mind-body component. Normalizing serum cholesterol levels addresses only one of the issues and often gives both doctors and patients an excuse for ignoring the others. (Fifty percent of people who suffer a first heart attack have normal serum cholesterol.) I'm not opposed to this kind of screening and treatment; I get it myself. I just have some concerns about it.

I am distinctly less enthusiastic about new, more complicated blood tests called "fractionated cholesterol screening" that give much more information about the types and subtypes of cholesterol and related lipids circulating in the blood. These tests are considerably more expensive and seem to me to give too much information, usually more than your doctor can interpret. As a result, they often create anxiety, especially since what to do about the management of abnormalities revealed by them may not be clear.

I am even more bothered by the widespread use of electron beam computed tomography (EBCT) scans of coronary arteries to reveal the amount of calcification in them, a test that exposes the body to radiation, is expensive and not covered by insurance, and is not endorsed by mainstream cardiologists. The problem here is that interpretation of results is not at all straightforward. A high calcium score may indicate increased risk of a coronary "event," such as a heart attack, but it may not. We know that atherosclerotic plaque becomes calcified and that rupture of a calcified plaque with a subsequent blood clot can obstruct a coronary artery, causing a heart attack. But the EBCT scan cannot show where the calcium is. Is it in the lining of the artery (more dangerous) or in the muscular wall (less dangerous)? Nor does it say how long the calcium has been there. It could be part of an old, stable plaque (less likely to rupture) or a new, unstable one (higher risk). Stable calcification of coronary arteries that has developed gradually over time may actually decrease the risk of heart attack in those with atherosclerosis.

The prospect of a noninvasive and accurate diagnostic test for coronary artery disease is appealing. It would be safer and cheaper than current angiographic techniques, and it may not be far off. Until then, I would be cautious about getting calcium scores and taking any drastic action based on them. Often, the use of EBCT to look at coronary arteries is part of a "total body scan," much in use by antiaging doctors, in which EBCT pictures are taken from head to toe. It has great potential to turn up abnormalities with no clinical significance, like nonspecific brain lesions. The main result is to make people more anxious about their bodies and get them to spend more money on more invasive tests.

The PSA (prostate-specific antigen) blood test, widely used to screen for prostate cancer in men, illustrates another kind of deficiency. It often gives false positives, but even when it does detect cancers, it gives no information about their nature—specifically, how aggressive they are and how likely they are to metastasize. That is really what we need to know, because most older men develop prostate cancer, and in most cases the risk of spread is low. A man can live to a ripe old age, enjoy good general health, and die with cancer contained in his prostate. The problem here is that a positive PSA test is often the first step down a road ending in radical prostatectomy, an operation that has many risks and may be completely unnecessary. Until we have a reliable follow-up test that can clearly distinguish aggressive from nonaggressive tumors, I have doubts about the wisdom of using the PSA as a general screening tool, except for those at high risk on the basis of family history and lifestyle.

On the other hand, I am strongly in favor of bone mineral density testing (the DEXA scan) for women at risk of osteoporosis. (Men can develop this bone-thinning disease, too, but usually much later in life than women.) If a woman knows her mother developed osteoporosis after menopause and she fits the profile of a person at risk (light boned, fair complexioned), she certainly should know her bone mineral density and how fast it is declining over time. Effective drug treatments are available to halt and reverse osteoporosis and so reduce risk of hip fracture, a major cause of disability and untimely death. Yet I also see unwise use of bone mineral density testing, because it allows us to identify and diagnose early cases of "osteopenia," or bone weakness, that are not anywhere near the range of serious osteoporosis. This is analogous to diagnosing "prehypertension," "prediabetes," and other very early stages of disease that may or may not progress and may be reversible by changing habits of diet, exercise, and other aspects of lifestyle. I have seen more women recently who have been told to start strong drugs to manage mild osteopenia—not good medicine in my judgment.

So how are you to decide how much of modern preventive medicine to use? I can only tell you to do your homework and be informed. Here are some general suggestions:

- Keep a personal medical record that includes information of past illnesses, injuries, treatments, hospitalizations, current medications, and family history. Based on family history, identify the categories of age-related disease you are most at risk for, such as cardiovascular disease, cancer, diabetes, and Alzheimer's disease, and know the preventive lifestyle strategies to keep them at bay.
- Make sure you have had recommended immunizations and have kept them current. Here is a Web site from the Centers for Disease Control and Prevention that gives this information: www.cdc.gov/nip/recs/adult-schedule.htm. I am very much in favor of immunization. Although I question the number of immunizations now being used in infants and children and the need for some of them (like those for chicken pox), I firmly believe that the benefits outweigh the risks. In addition to the immunizations given in early life, those sixty-five and older should get pneumococcal pneumonia vaccine and an annual influenza shot.
- Get a complete physical examination that includes measurement of blood pressure, urinalysis, and complete blood work, as well as an electrocardiogram (EKG). This will screen for such common conditions as hypertension, diabetes, elevated serum cholesterol, anemia, and liver or kidney problems. Keep the results in your personal medical record. I do not necessarily recommend annual medical examinations if you are in good health and have no unusual symptoms. Discuss with your health-care provider how often to have them.
- Learn about recommended screening tests appropriate

for your age. A good place to start is the Web site of the National Women's Health Information Center (www.4woman.gov/screeningcharts/general.htm), which also has recommendations for men (www.4woman.gov/screeningcharts/mens.htm). This site gives details about Pap smears and mammograms for women, colonoscopies for all persons, and bone mineral density testing. It does not recommend total body scans or calcium scoring of coronary arteries, and I am pleased that it deals with the PSA test for men by saying, "Discuss with your health-care provider." Please remember, however, that it is your responsibility to inform yourself about the pros and cons of all diagnostic tests.

- Maintain blood pressure in the normal range—that is, 120/80 or below. If your blood pressure is *consistently* elevated, even when you measure it yourself, first try to normalize it by changing your habits of diet, exercise, and relaxation. If that fails, use medication, starting with a low dose of a mild agent.
- In general, if you are diagnosed with a precondition, such as prehypertension or prediabetes, first try to reverse it by nonpharmacological means. If that doesn't work, use the mildest medication available at the lowest effective dose.

A great deal of information is available in books, newsletters, and Web sites about self-care and healthy living. I recommend some of them in Appendix B. I also advise you to read my books *Natural Health, Natural Medicine* and *8 Weeks to Optimum Health* (both recently revised and updated), which give detailed practical suggestions for maintaining health and managing common ailments on your own, using natural methods when possible. I am not going to repeat all of that material here, but I do want to discuss a few specific points of preventive health care that need emphasis before I give you my advice about what the body needs if it is to enjoy healthy aging:

- *Don't smoke.* Tobacco addiction is the single greatest cause of preventable illness, and tobacco smoke is the most obvious environmental cause of cancer. Yes, there are centenarians and other very old people who smoke and have done so for most of their lives. They are blessed (or cursed) with genes that allow them to detoxify the harmful combustion products of tobacco. Most people do not have that genetic protection and are at much greater risk. Exposure to tobacco smoke not only increases the odds of developing many kinds of cancer, it also raises the risks of cardiovascular and respiratory diseases that are simply incompatible with healthy aging. Inhalation of vaporized nicotine is as addictive as the smoking of crack cocaine or crystal methamphetamine. Almost all cases of tobacco addiction begin in the teenage years or earlier; therefore, I address this message to young readers. Do not experiment with smoking: the chance of becoming addicted is too great, and this is one of the hardest of all addictions to break. Young women may be more susceptible than young men at the moment, because smoking appeals to them as a method of appetite suppression and weight control.
- *Watch your weight.* Morbid obesity, sometimes defined as being more than a hundred pounds above one's "normal" weight, is incompatible with healthy aging, because it increases the risk of a number of age-related diseases, including cardiovascular disease, type 2 diabetes, and osteoarthritis, that often lead to premature disability and death. Ordinary obesity—weighing at least 20 percent

more than you should—correlates with milder forms of those diseases as well as with increased incidence of post-menopausal breast cancer and cancer of the uterus, colon, kidney, and esophagus. But what is normal and how much should you weigh?

With so much publicity about the obesity epidemic in North America, people have become obsessed with weight and dieting. Fad diets are more popular than ever, bogus products claiming to promote weight loss are ubiquitous, and bariatric (weight-management) medicine has become a booming specialty. But we are tempted by more and more fattening foods in great abundance, even while the fashion and entertainment industries continue to promote anorexic leanness as the ideal of attractiveness and sexuality. No wonder people are driven crazy about their weight.

Sorting out the medical realities about weight is not so easy. It is quite possible that our criteria for obesity and our thinking about its medical implications have been warped by fashion. We all know morbid obesity when we see it; clearly, it interferes with activities of daily living and makes people unhappy, unhealthy, and unlikely to experience successful aging. But is that true of simply being overweight, as indicated by tables of ideal heights and weights and measurements of BMI, the body mass index?

I don't think so. In fact, being too lean may also compromise health and successful aging. I will have more to say about that later, when I discuss physical activity. Here I will note that those who are somewhat overweight in middle age may enjoy a healthier and longer old age than those who are not and state my belief that it is better to be fit and fat than lean and not fit.

What that means is that if you are somewhat overweight and cannot maintain the ideal weight of actuarial tables, you should concentrate on maintaining optimum health by eating right and keeping physically active. I will give you detailed advice on how to do that in the following chapters.

Finally, I want to say some further words to younger readers. First of all, the earlier in life you start to think about how you want to age and start doing something about it, the better. I'm not going to take the time to tell you why you should wear seat belts when you ride in cars and floss your teeth after meals; you can find that information elsewhere. I will warn you about accidents, violence, and suicide, the common pitfalls for the young. If you like adrenaline highs, please be careful about how you get them. Seek out experienced guides if you engage in hazardous activities, whether it be skydiving, rock climbing, extreme sports, using drugs and alcohol, or experimenting with sex. Know the hazards of the activities you choose and know how to contain them.

If you spend time with people who are violent, put yourself in violent situations, or otherwise feed the propensity for violence that is part of human nature, you are likely to get hurt or worse. Enough said. As for suicide, the rate of it is rising in children, adolescents, and young adults, and it is often linked to depression and low self-esteem. These problems are identifiable and treatable. Do not hesitate to seek professional help if you have them. See Chapter 15 for more information about mental and emotional health and their impact on how we age.

9

BODY II: THE ANTI-INFLAMMATORY DIET

Throughout life the need for good nutrition is a constant. I have written a great deal about diet and health in other books.* I have also taught classes and seminars on this topic and organized large continuing-education conferences on it for health professionals. Still, I feel it is necessary to say more. Contemporary eating habits are cause for great concern. Fast food has replaced meals cooked at home. Refined and processed foods fill the shelves of supermarkets. People jump from one fad diet to the next. And health-care professionals are not much help, because their education in nutrition, if any, was inadequate.

At the same time, the science of nutrition is developing rapidly. Pick up any medical journal, and you will find articles reporting results of studies of the influence of specific foods or components of foods on health. The scientific facts are there; they just don't make it into medical school cur-

---

*Natural Health, Natural Medicine, rev. ed. (Boston: Houghton Mifflin, 2004); 8 Weeks to Optimum Health, rev ed. (New York: Knopf, 2006); Eating Well for Optimum Health (New York: Alfred A. Knopf, 2000); The Healthy Kitchen (with Rosie Daley) (New York: Alfred A. Knopf, 2002).

riculums, leaving doctors functionally illiterate in this most important field of knowledge and unable to help patients make sense of the confusing and often contradictory information in the media and in the marketplace.

Most books about nutrition that cross my desk are diet books, intended to help people lose weight. It should be obvious by now that diets don't work, except in the short term. By definition, diets are regimens that you go off of, and when people go off them, lost weight is almost always regained. The main predictor of success with any diet is whether people stick to it. You can lose weight on a low-fat diet or a low-carbohydrate diet or any other sort of restrictive eating plan if you stay on it; you will regain weight if you don't. Many popular fad diets will do you no harm over a few weeks, but some can undermine health in the long term.

I am going to urge you to follow a diet that I believe can increase the probability of healthy aging, but I hesitate even to call it a diet. It is absolutely not intended as a weight-loss program, nor is it an eating plan to stay on for a limited period of time. Rather, it is the nutritional component of a healthy lifestyle, a way of selecting and preparing foods based on scientific knowledge of how they can help your body resist and adapt to the changes that time brings. I refer to it as a diet only because people are so hungry for rules and plans about eating. I like to call it the Anti-inflammatory Diet. If you want to think of it as a longevity diet, feel free to do so, but remember that the goal is compression of morbidity, not life extension.

Earlier, I referred to inflammation as a common root of many chronic diseases and wrote about oxidative stress as a proinflammatory influence. Before I can explain the Anti-inflammatory Diet, I want to be sure that you have a clear understanding of the inflammatory process and its role in health and disease. So permit me to restate and expand on what I wrote earlier.

The word "inflammation" suggests "fire within," a graphic if inaccurate image of what happens when the four classic symptoms and signs of inflammation appear. They are, in the original Latin learned by medical students, *rubor, calor, turgor,* and *dolor*—that is, redness, heat, swelling, and pain. Think about an immediate injury to the skin, from an impact or a burn. Think about an infected finger or toe. Think about a "hot" joint. In all such cases, those four changes occur together. They announce that a part of the body is inflamed.

Heat and redness represent an influx of blood to the area. Swelling comes from changes in the walls of small blood vessels that allow plasma to seep into tissues. Pain results from the release of messenger compounds used by the immune system to draw defensive support to an area that is injured or under assault. We perceive these changes as unpleasant. They draw attention to the affected part of the body and may interfere with normal activity and rest. But inflammation is visible evidence of the body's healing system at work. It marks the arrival of nourishment and immune activity in an area that needs them. Ordinarily, the signs and symptoms of inflammation should be welcomed, not shunned.

Then why do we try to counteract inflammation with anti-inflammatory drugs and herbs? Why should we consider an anti-inflammatory diet? The answer requires a distinction between normal and abnormal inflammation. The normal process is a central aspect of healing, absolutely necessary and desirable in the defense, maintenance, and repair of the body, both inside and outside, throughout life. Normal inflammation is the healing system's response to localized injury and attack. It is confined to that location, serves a purpose, and ends when the problem resolves. Any discomfort or limitation of function it causes is the price to be paid for healing.

Abnormal inflammation extends beyond its appointed limits in space and time. It spreads to areas of the body that have not experienced injury or attack, and it does not end when the problem that elicited it resolves. The inflammatory process unleashes some of the immune system's most sophisticated weaponry, including enzymes that can rupture cell walls and digest vital components of cells and tissues. Like military weapons, they can be equally damaging to both friend and foe. The destructive potential of inflammation is so great that the body must control the process tightly, confining it in space and time and turning it off when it has achieved its purpose. When inflammation escapes this control, when it targets normal tissues, when it just won't quit, it is abnormal and promotes disease rather than healing.

One broad category of disease marked by unchecked inflammation is autoimmunity. When the immune system attacks the body's own tissues for no good reason, a condition of autoimmunity exists that can cause discomfort, disability, failure of organs, and sometimes irreparable damage to vital structures. Type 1 diabetes is autoimmune in origin; abnormal immune attack, triggered by an unknown cause, usually early in life, destroys the insulin-producing cells of the pancreas. Before the availability of insulin replacement, a diagnosis of type 1 diabetes usually meant an early death. Rheumatic fever is autoimmune: in some susceptible people a streptococcus infection of the throat can trigger the immune system to attack the joints and heart valves. Before the availability of penicillin to treat strep infections, rheumatic fever was much more common and a frequent cause of rheumatic heart disease from scarring of the delicate tissue of the valves. Rheumatoid arthritis and systemic lupus erythematasus are autoimmune. Autoimmunity can target the liver, the brain, the muscles, and the skin. It can be a component of other diseases, like multiple sclerosis and inflammatory bowel disease. Infection, toxic injury, and stress can all initiate autoimmune reactions in susceptible people, though in many cases the triggers are unknown. Whatever the trigger, the damage caused by autoimmunity has an obvious immediate cause: inappropriate, unchecked inflammation.

When I was in medical school, I was taught that the primary problem in asthma was bronchoconstriction: tightening of the small airways in the chest. The main treatment offered was medication to dilate those airways. The current conception of asthma is very different. It is now viewed as an inflammatory disorder of the airways, with bronchoconstriction secondary to the irritation caused by inflammation. Anti-inflammatory drugs, such as inhaled steroids, are now mainstays of treatment. Asthma is increasing in frequency all over the world, for reasons that are not clear. Worsening air pollution probably contributes, but asthma is as much on the increase in areas with clean air as elsewhere. Might some other environmental change be promoting inflammation?

Until quite recently, the root cause of coronary heart disease was thought to be atherosclerosis, deposits of cholesterol in artery walls as a result of elevated cholesterol levels in the blood. The consensus among cardiologists today is that inflammation of the lining of arteries is more of a root cause. Deposits of cholesterol may even be a flawed healing response of the body, an attempt to patch defects caused by inflammatory damage. A new blood test to measure

C-reactive protein has received much attention from cardiologists as a predictor of heart attack risk; elevated levels indicate active inflammation in arteries. Why do so many people in our part of the world develop this problem?

Alzheimer's disease is marked by structural changes in the brain—tangles of filaments within nerve cells and accumulations of plaques of an unusual protein outside them. No one knows where these abnormal structures come from, but inflammation in the brain seems to precede their appearance, and anti-inflammatory drugs like ibuprofen reduce the risk of developing this devastating and incurable neurodegenerative disease. Other diseases in this category—ALS and Parkinson's disease, for example—may also share a component of abnormal inflammation. One neurologist who specializes in their prevention and treatment emphasizes this aspect of neurodegenerative disease by using the phrase "brain on fire."

Even some of the so-called functional diseases—those that can cause real suffering but without any objective changes in body structures that doctors can document—may be linked. One example is irritable bowel syndrome (IBS), marked by variable degrees of abdominal pain, constipation or diarrhea, and abdominal bloating. New research suggests that microinflammation may be occurring throughout the GI tract—patchy areas of tissue damage visible only on microscopic examination.

Asthma and autoimmune disorders often appear in childhood or youth, but many diseases now associated with abnormal inflammation become much more frequent as people grow older. Coronary heart disease and neurodegenerative diseases are broad categories of age-related disease, just the sorts of conditions we should be trying to avoid if we are to enjoy healthy aging.

Except for relatively rare childhood cancers and some

leukemias and lymphomas, the vast majority of malignancies appear in people sixty and older. Cancer is a classic age-related disease, one that can drastically interfere with quality of life and cause premature death. It has always been placed in a class by itself, called *neoplastic* disease, because it involves the growth of new tissue, and we never thought it had anything in common with chronic degenerative diseases. But now, with the focus of medical attention on abnormal inflammation, some scientists are beginning to sketch a connection.

The complex and precise regulation of the inflammatory process is under the control of hormones, such as prostaglandins and leukotrienes. Like most regulatory molecules, these come in families with opposite effects. Some upregulate (intensify) inflammatory activity, while others downregulate (dampen) it. In order for normal inflammation to serve the healing process and not become abnormal and productive of disease, these regulating hormones must be in equilibrium, responding both to the body's needs for defensive action and to disturbing influences on it from without. The relevant fact here is that the same hormones that upregulate inflammation also stimulate cells to proliferate, while those that downregulate it have an opposite action. Whenever cells divide more frequently, the risk of malignant transformation increases. Therefore, anything that promotes inflammation through a hormonal mechanism also has the potential to promote the development of cancer.

Here is the beginning of a radically new and exciting hypothesis about age-related disease. Much of it may be the result of abnormal inflammation or abnormal activity of the hormones that promote inflammation. I use the word "exciting" because this way of thinking opens up new and relatively simple ways of modifying or preventing this common cause of large categories of disease that are the main barriers to healthy aging.

I believe without question that diet influences inflammation. The food choices we make can determine whether we are in a pro-inflammatory state or an anti-inflammatory one. In the former case, abnormal inflammation is more likely, as are all the diseases associated with it. In the latter case, normal inflammation is unaffected; that is, the body's healing responses to injury and infection are as they should be, and the risks of disease caused by abnormal inflammation remain low as we age. The ways that diet and inflammatory status interplay are myriad. I can give you a sense of this by walking you through the categories of nutrients we need.

We need macronutrients in relatively large amounts as sources of energy and materials to maintain and repair tissues. They are fats, carbohydrates, and proteins, and they all affect inflammatory status in different ways. Micronutrients are substances we need in much smaller amounts for optimal functioning of the body; they include vitamins, minerals, fiber, and phytonutrients. The last are plant-derived compounds that are the objects of a great deal of research attention, because of their powerful impact on health. Micronutrients, especially phytonutrients, can also influence whether we go through life inflamed or not.

The most obvious dietary connection to inflammation and the one that has been most publicized concerns fats. The body synthesizes prostaglandins and leukotrienes from polyunsaturated fatty acids (PUFAs), which are essential nutrients. "Essential" means that our bodies can't make them and we have to get them from our food. We need two classes of PUFAs, omega-3 and omega-6 fatty acids, and we require them regularly and in proper ratio. In general, the hormones synthesized from omega-6 fatty acids upregulate inflammation, while those made from omega-3s have an opposite effect. Omega-6s are widely available in the diet in oil-rich seeds and the vegetable oils extracted from them. They also build up in the fat of grain-fed animals we eat.

For example, arachidonic acid, originally found in peanut oil (*Arachis* is the botanical name of the peanut), is a significant constituent of chicken fat. It is the starting point of a biochemical pathway first described by Sir John Vane, who won the 1982 Nobel Prize for medicine for his elucidation of the therapeutic effect of aspirin. He showed that aspirin and related anti-inflammatory drugs worked by inhibiting enzymes that convert arachidonic acid to pro-inflammatory hormones. The arachidonic acid pathway is the biochemical route to increased inflammation, but remember that inflammation is the central component of the body's immune defenses and healing system. The arachidonic acid pathway is a necessary element of human biochemistry. It leads to problems only when its activity is out of balance with that of the synthesis of anti-inflammatory hormones.

Unfortunately, the starting materials for the anti-inflammatory pathway, the omega-3s, are much harder to come by. They occur in low concentrations in leafy greens, a few seeds and nuts (walnuts, flax, hemp), a few vegetable oils (soy, canola), sea vegetables, and oily fish from cold waters (salmon, sardines, herring, mackerel, black cod [sablefish], bluefish). Animals that are allowed to graze on grass rather than being fattened on grains accumulate omega-3s in their fat.

Many authorities on nutrition believe that the ratio of omega-6 to omega-3 fatty acids in the human diet was roughly equal in the distant past and has become more and more unequal in modern diets, especially in industrialized

Western countries, where people now consume far more omega-6s than omega-3s. Reasons for this change in ratio include the flooding of today's diet with refined vegetable oils, products of modern food technology; the practice of fattening food animals, especially cows, on grain; increased consumption of meat relative to fish; and decreased consumption of greens and other vegetable sources of omega-3s. If you go into any American supermarket or convenience store, almost all of the snack foods you will find there— all of the chips, crackers, cookies, and candy—provide omega-6 fatty acids and no omega-3s. Most fast food is rich in omega-6s and devoid of omega-3s. (In the past few years, fish consumption has increased as people have learned of its health benefits, but I think that trend may now change, with so much publicity about mercury and other toxins in many species of fish, including, sadly, some of the best omega-3 sources.)

The two diets most associated with longevity and compression of morbidity—the traditional Japanese diet and the Mediterranean diet—are both notable for their favorable omega-3 to omega-6 ratio, the result of the inclusion of fish, emphasis on vegetables (including sea vegetables in Japanese cuisine), exclusion of refined and processed foods made with vegetable oils, and minimal reliance on meat. By contrast, most North Americans and Europeans are deficient in omega-3s, a dietary imbalance that may account for the rise of such diseases as asthma, coronary heart disease, many forms of cancer, autoimmunity, and neurodegenerative disease.

And the omega-6 to omega-3 ratio is only part of the story of how fats influence inflammation. Some fats are distinctly proinflammatory and, in my view, have no place in any diet intended to promote healthy aging. They are the artificially hardened fats: margarine, vegetable shortening, and partially hydrogenated vegetable oils. The processing that turns liquid oils into semisolid fats deforms them chemically, resulting in products that directly increase inflammation and may over time push the body into a pro-inflammatory state. These products include oxidized fatty acids and trans fats. Liquid oils are unsaturated, as opposed to solid (saturated) fats like lard and butter. Unsaturation means that the oils are rich in fatty acid molecules containing double and triple bonds between carbon atoms. These bonds are points of instability that are vulnerable to attack by oxygen and that can spring into unnatural positions—creating trans fats—if the oils are heated or otherwise disturbed. Oxidized fatty acids account for the rancidity of oils exposed to air, light, and heat. Trans fats are not detectable by our noses, but they are sure to be present in any products made with partially hydrogenated oils.

To avoid consuming these unhealthy fats, you just need to follow some simple rules:

- Do not eat any products listing partially hydrogenated oil as an ingredient, regardless of the type of oil.
- Do not use vegetable shortening (e.g., Crisco) or products made with it.
- New regulations in the United States will require listing of the trans fat content of foods. If you follow the first two rules above, you do not have to worry about trans fats.
- Do not eat margarine, regardless of what it is made from or what health benefits manufacturers claim for it. Use butter, olive oil, or natural butter substitutes that are made semisolid by the mechanical process of emulsification rather than the chemical process of hydrogenation.
- Avoid fried food in restaurants, especially fast-food restaurants. The oils in the fryers will contain oxidized fats.

- Train your nose to detect rancidity: it's the smell of oil paint (oxidized linseed [flax] oil). Throw out any oils that smell rancid. Do not eat any nuts, seeds, or whole-grain flours or cereals that smell rancid. Smell any commercial products made with oil to check for rancidity before you eat them.

- Minimize the use of polyunsaturated vegetable oils, such as safflower, sunflower, corn, sesame, and soy. They are more likely to oxidize and go rancid than monounsaturated oils like olive and canola. (High-oleic safflower oil and high-oleic sunflower oils are okay; they are patented products, from strains of these plants that produce oils with better fatty-acid profiles, closer in composition to olive oil.) Buy oils in smaller rather than larger quantities. Protect them from exposure to air, light, and heat, and use them up quickly. (Refrigerate them if you can't.) It is fine to use nut oils in unheated preparations like salad dressings and roasted (dark) sesame oil in small amounts as a flavoring.

- Never heat oils to the point of smoking. Never reuse oils that have been heated to high temperatures. Never breathe the smoke of oils heated to high temperatures.

- Most vegetable oils in the supermarket are extracted with heat and solvents that create undesirable chemical changes and pro-inflammatory products. Use expeller- or cold-pressed oils. Use extra-virgin olive oil; other kinds, like "light" olive oil, have been chemically refined and are not as healthy.

In Appendix A, you will find a complete summary of the Anti-inflammatory Diet, with specific recommendations for foods to include and foods to avoid. Here I just want you to understand the general influences of diet on the inflammatory process, beginning with the very important role of fats and oils. In a nutshell: you can reduce the risks of abnormal inflammation and diseases associated with it and shift your body from a pro-inflammatory to an anti-inflammatory state by increasing your intake of omega-3 fatty acids, decreasing your intake of omega-6 fatty acids, and excluding from your diet the kinds of fats known to promote inflammation.

Most people I talk to these days have some familiarity with the information just presented. Fewer are aware of the influence of carbohydrate choices on inflammatory status. The connection is easy to grasp; I described it earlier when I discussed the glycation theory of aging. Remember that "glycation" is the name of chemical reactions between sugars and proteins that account for the browning of foods. When these reactions occur in the human body, they produce pro-inflammatory compounds that have been termed AGEs for advanced glycation end products. AGEs can directly promote inflammation. They can also deform proteins by cross-linking them; cross-linked proteins can further promote inflammation. Therefore, you want to minimize the amount of glycation going on in your body.

Doctors treating patients with diabetes measure glycation to monitor the severity of the disease and the effectiveness of measures to control it. They do so by checking blood levels of hemoglobin A1C, a form of glycated hemoglobin. Hemoglobin is the oxygen-carrying pigment protein in red blood cells. It can react with glucose in the blood to form a stable sugar-protein complex, hemoglobin A1C. Blood sugar levels fluctuate greatly and frequently, affected by the digestion of food, physical activity, stress, and other factors. Whenever they are high, glycation of hemoglobin occurs. Once hemoglobin A1C is formed, it persists in the body until the red blood cells carrying it are eliminated; the normal life span of red blood cells is 90 to 120 days. Therefore the amount of hemoglobin A1C in the blood gives an indication of mean blood glucose over the past three months, a much more meaningful indicator of the amount of sugar floating around the system than any number of blood glucose measurements.

Moreover, it reveals the amount of glycation going on throughout the body, which is what you really want to know, because that process affects other proteins and generates AGEs. It is the products of glycation that cause many of the pathological changes that occur in diabetes if the disease is not controlled. I have written that diabetes provides a model of accelerated aging and suggests the importance of the insulin system as a determinant of how we age. Instead of the compression of morbidity we should all be aiming for, diabetics are at risk for expansion of morbidity, with age-related diseases appearing much earlier in life than they should. Glycation is responsible, and whenever blood sugar is elevated, glycation is occurring.

Now, normal people have low levels of hemoglobin A1C. In fact, the upper limit of normal is set at 6 percent of total hemoglobin. Amounts greater than that suggest prediabetes or frank diabetes, requiring lifestyle modifications or medications to keep blood sugar in the normal range more of the time. As with oxidative stress, we have defense mechanisms to protect us from the low level of glycation resulting from normal processing of food and distribution of caloric energy.

The thrifty genes described earlier predispose many of us to develop "metabolic syndromes" marked by disturbances in these systems. Metabolic syndromes come in many forms and degrees, ranging from slight abnormalities in blood lipids, borderline hypertension, and a tendency to gain weight easily, especially in the abdomen, to prediabetes at the other extreme. The common theme in these syndromes is insulin resistance. Cells lose insulin receptors, and the pancreas tries to overcome the deficit by pumping out more of the hormone. Meanwhile, sugar levels in the blood spike, especially after consumption of quickly digested carbohydrate foods, and those levels stay elevated longer than they should. Eating too many calories, eating the wrong kinds of carbohydrate foods, and lack of physical activity put people with metabolic syndromes at risk for obesity and type 2 diabetes, but even before those problems appear, frequent spiking of blood sugar will favor glycation and its long-term detrimental effects on health. It may be that half the population or more has this genetic heritage. And even those without it would do well to learn the difference between quickly digested and slowly digested carbohydrates, because eating fewer of the former and more of the latter is better for optimum health. The quickly digested ones are often low-quality foods that should not be prominent in a diet for healthy aging.

That difference is measured on a scale called the glycemic index (GI) that ranges from zero to 100, with glucose at the top. Foods rated 70 and above are considered high-GI carbohydrates that have a fast and strong influence on blood sugar; those between 55 and 70 are moderate; and those below 55 are low. Currently, a new scale, the glycemic load (GL), is gaining more acceptance. It factors in the actual amount of carbohydrate consumed in a portion of a given food and is more accurate than GI alone.

Glycemic load addresses the problem that some foods, like carrots and beets, score high on the GI scale but actually have only a modest load of carbohydrate, diluted by fiber and water. Proponents of low-carbohydrate diets who look only at the GI tell people never to let carrots or beets cross their lips. But if you calculate the glycemic load of these vegetables (GI multiplied by the grams of carbohydrate in a serving), they both score in the low to moderate range. Low GL values are 1–10; moderate, 11–19; and high, 20 and up. You can learn more about these concepts and look up GI and GL values for many foods on the Internet.*

Here are some general recommendations for choosing carbohydrate sources wisely to minimize abnormal inflammation:

- Become informed about glycemic index and glycemic load. Ignore obsolete information that classifies carbohydrates as simple and complex.
- Reduce consumption of high-GL foods, replacing them with low- to moderate-GL foods. That means less bread, white potatoes, crackers, chips and other snack foods, pastries, and sweetened drinks and more whole grains, beans, sweet potatoes, winter squashes, and other vegetables. Eat temperate fruits (berries, cherries, apples, pears) in moderation, rather than tropical fruits (pineapple, mango, papaya).
- Eat less refined and processed food.
- Eat less fast food, or, better, avoid it altogether.
- Eat fewer products made with flour of any kind.
- Avoid products made with high-fructose corn syrup.

You will find more detailed recommendations about carbohydrate foods in Appendix A.

*Three sites I use are www.diabetes.about.com/library/mendosagi/ngilists.htm; http://lpi.oregonstate.edu/infocenter/foods/grains/gigl.html; and www.harvard.edu/hhp/article/content.do?name=WNO104d.

Proteins are the third category of macronutrients. Their influence on inflammatory status is not as direct as that of fats and carbohydrates, because it has to do less with the protein itself than with what comes along with it.

For example, most protein foods contain fat, and the fat can be pro-inflammatory (chicken) or anti-inflammatory (oily fish). (Also, animal fat is mostly saturated, and diets high in saturated fat increase the risks of atherosclerosis and cardiovascular disease by their influence on cholesterol production.) In addition, protein foods come with greater or lesser amounts of environmental toxins. In general, foods of animal origin are more contaminated than plant foods, because animals are higher up on the food chain, the sequence of organisms in which those above feed on those below. At every step up the food chain there is a greater chance of accumulating and concentrating toxins found in the environment. Toxic load can tip the human body's balance toward an inflammatory state as well as undermine its defenses.

This is not necessarily an argument for becoming a vegan or a vegetarian, but it does suggest that it is a good idea to reduce consumption of meat and other animal protein and increase consumption of vegetable protein, such as soy and other legumes. Vegetable protein comes with fewer toxins and with healthier fat; often, it provides beneficial phytonutrients as well.

Fish deserves special comment. For years, I have recommended eating more fish, especially in place of meat, both for its high-quality protein and for associated omega-3 fatty acids in species like salmon and sardines. But in the past few years, I have become increasingly concerned about the dangerous levels of mercury and PCBs and other organic toxins in many of the fish we eat, both wild and farmed. In my own diet, I still include wild Alaskan salmon, Alaskan black cod (sablefish or butterfish), and sardines as omega-3 sources, but I also take a daily dose of fish oil (distilled and toxin free), and recommend that to people who cannot get wild Alaskan fish and do not like canned sardines. Occasionally in restaurants I eat other fish, like haddock and Pacific cod, but I am very selective.

You should know that the toxic content of many popular fish—tuna and halibut, for example—depends on size: the bigger the fish, the more mercury and PCBs it's going to have. Some suppliers are buying up and selling small tuna and halibut, which the big distributors don't want. If you like these fish, try to eat small ones only—say in the ten-to-fifteen-pound range. Farmed salmon presents a tough problem. It is more available and cheaper than wild salmon and is now everywhere. It looks good and tastes good to most people. Salmon farmers are capable of producing fish that are relatively free of toxins and can even bring the omega-3 content up to equal or exceed that of wild salmon. It's all a matter of providing the right kind of clean feed. Until consumers demand that, however, salmon farmers are not going to change their ways. In the meantime, you should know that sockeye (red) salmon is the one variety that cannot yet be farmed, meaning that all sockeye salmon you see in markets and in cans is wild. I recommend it.

So, for the role of protein in the Anti-inflammatory Diet, my advice is simple:

- Eat less meat and poultry and other foods of animal origin.
- Eat more vegetable protein: soy foods, other legumes (beans, lentils), whole grains, seeds, and nuts.

- If you eat fish, choose only varieties and sources that are likely to carry the fewest toxic contaminants.

That brings us to the micronutrients. Vitamins and minerals in the right amounts support healthy immune function. We get most of them by eating fruits and vegetables, which also provide fiber and phytonutrients. It is this last group of compounds that is of most interest to me in considering the inflammatory status of the body. I discuss dietary supplements in the next chapter. Here I will comment on some of the plant compounds that I think have the most important protective effects, the ones that should be included in any diet for healthy aging.

The general rule is simply to eat more fruits and vegetables. These foods are prominent in the Mediterranean and traditional Japanese diets, much more so than in typical diets of western Europe and North America. We are now told to eat seven or more servings of fruits and vegetables a day, but we are usually given no information about the kinds and quality of produce to look for. I believe it is important to eat as many fresh fruits and vegetables as possible and, as with protein foods, to learn to select those that are least likely to be contaminated with toxins.

A colleague of mine, Dr. David Heber, director of the Center for Studies of Human Nutrition at the University of California, Los Angeles, has written a book entitled *What Color Is Your Diet?* He urges readers to include produce from all parts of the color spectrum in order to get the full range of protective phytonutrients. Many of the pigments that plants pack into their fruits, leaves, stems, and roots are key parts of their defensive systems, including defenses against oxidative stress. Heber sorts plant foods into seven colors, all with different healthful properties: red, red-purple, orange, orange-yellow, yellow-green, green, and white-green. He suggests that we avoid the white and beige snack foods and processed foods made from refined grains that have bad fats and carbohydrates and are not sources of phytonutrients. Instead, we should "colorize" our diets in order to protect our DNA. Heber recommends at least one serving a day—that is, one-half cup cooked or one cup raw—of a fruit or vegetable from each color group. That would be quite a stretch for people eating main-stream North American diets, but I think it is a good goal to aim for.

Let's take a look at just two large families of plant pigments, those accounting for reds and purples and those creating oranges and yellows. The first are the anthocyanins, the second the carotenoids.

Once considered waste products in plant tissues, anthocyanins are now regarded as having important roles in maintaining the health of plants that make them and of animals that eat the plants. Over three hundred have been discovered, all water soluble. They occur in distinctive groupings that give each plant species a particular pigment "fingerprint." For example, red wine contains fifteen of these compounds, the varying proportions of which determine the wine's color and indicate the type of grapes that went into it. Anthocyanins often occur in high concentrations in young shoots and leaves, like the red leaves of maple trees in early spring. This is a clue to one of their biological functions. They absorb visible and ultraviolet light to minimize oxidative damage induced by solar radiation in vulnerable young tissue and are highly protective against other kinds of stress as well. An interesting fact to surface recently is that plants under environmental stress increase production of anthocyanins. Organically grown fruits and vegetables experience more environmental stress, as from insect predation, and as a result they contain more of these pigments. This is an early bit of evidence supporting the long-standing claim of organic growers that their produce is more nutritious, a claim long disputed by conventional nutritionists and plant scientists.

The International Workshop on Anthocyanins held in Sydney, Australia, in January 2004 drew scientists from many countries and gave an indication of how much research is now under way on this subject. In a preface to the program, the workshop chairpersons wrote:

> Anthocyanin-rich fruit and vegetable extracts evaluated in both *in vitro* and *in vivo* experimental systems demonstrated protection against oxidative damage caused by free radicals. Anthocyanins have been reported to provide protection against liver injuries and UV radiation, significantly reduce blood pressure, improve eyesight, exhibit strong anti-inflammatory and antimicrobial activities . . . and suppress proliferation of human cancer cells. Due to their wide physiological activities, anthocyanins may play a significant role in preventing lifestyle related diseases such as cancer, diabetes, and cardiovascular and neurological diseases.

When maple leaves turn green as spring advances, the anthocyanins are still there but are masked by chlorophyll. When chlorophyll production stops with the onset of cold weather in autumn, they and other pigments shine forth in the glory of fall foliage. In the same way, these colorful phytonutrients are present in dark leafy greens, like Swiss chard, kale, and collards; we just don't see them. Some of the best sources are berries, including blueberries, blackberries, and raspberries, and these have the added advantage of being fruits low on the glycemic load scale, so you can eat them freely. You may have read articles promoting blueberries as having specific antiaging effects. As far as I can determine, these are mostly part of a public-relations campaign of the Michigan Blueberry Growers Association. Nevertheless, I agree that blueberries are an excellent source of phytonutrients that can reduce risks of age-related disease and that do not cause unwanted spikes in blood sugar. They also occupy a narrow slice of the color spectrum that Dr. Heber does not mention. How many other blue foods can you think of? I eat blueberries frequently and always buy organic varieties.

That does not mean that you should gobble up blueberry jam or pie or blueberry muffins. In the presence of high sugar concentrations, anthocyanins are rapidly destroyed; therefore blueberry jam and pie filling are far less valuable sources than raw blueberries or blueberries cooked with little or no added sugar. Blueberry muffins have too few of the fruits relative to the amounts of white flour, sugar, and fat (usually saturated) they contain.

Besides berries, cherries, red grapes (and juice and wine made from them), and pomegranates (and their juice, which is increasingly available), red cabbage and beets are good sources of anthocyanins. Let your eyes guide you to these good foods, but don't forget the dark, leafy greens, best eaten lightly cooked.

Before I leave the subject of anthocyanins, I should mention that they are a subgroup of a larger class of plant compounds called flavonoids, and they, in turn, are a subclass of plant polyphenols, compounds with significant antioxidant activity, now being studied for their cancer-protective potential. You have heard about polyphenols in tea. The most important, EGCG (epigallocatechin gallate), is one of the most potent antioxidants known, responsible for many of the health benefits of tea reported in studies from Asia, Europe, and North America. I am a devotee of good tea and would like to write a few words about its place in the Anti-inflammatory Diet before going on to the orange and yellow sections of the food color spectrum.

All true tea comes from one plant species, *Camellia sinensis,* a relative of ornamental camellias. Herbal teas are not true tea, nor is rooibos tea from South Africa, often called red tea. These may have medicinal properties of their own, but they do not contain EGCG or the other polyphenols that make true tea so valuable. There are five recognized forms of tea that differ in color, flavor, and polyphenol content, depending on how the leaves are harvested and processed. Processing mostly involves exposing freshly picked leaves to air and heat before drying and packing them. This results in varying degrees of oxidation of the leaves (inaccurately called "fermentation" in many publications). Oxidation darkens color, intensifies flavor and creates new flavor elements, and degrades the polyphenol content. All tea has health benefits, but the less oxidized forms deliver more antioxidant activity and probably greater health-protective effects.

The least processed form is white tea from parts of China. Often quite expensive, it brews into a beverage that is almost colorless or very pale and has a most delicate flavor. Next on the scale is green tea, which comes in many varieties and qualities from places as diverse as India, China, and, of course, Japan. It is somewhat lower in antioxidant activity, stronger in color and flavor. Next is oolong tea, produced in quantity on the island of Taiwan and on mainland China. Intermediate in color, flavor, and antioxidant activity between green and black tea, it ranges from inexpensive, forgettable forms (Chinese restaurant tea) to exquisite brews that are the most expensive teas in the world, $10,000 a pound and more. Black tea, produced in great quantities in India, Ceylon, and Argentina, has been the form most familiar to Westerners. It is what we get in ordinary tea bags (usually the cheapest stuff of all) and what North Americans consume as iced tea. Finally, there is the curious *pu-erh* tea of China, very dark in color, with flavor notes of earth and tobacco and the least antioxidant activity. When brewed it can resemble coffee, and a tea importer friend of mine thinks it's the best form to use when trying to persuade coffee drinkers to switch to a healthier caffeinated drink.

I recommend drinking tea, especially white, green, and oolong, regularly—up to four cups a day. If you don't want all that caffeine or are very sensitive to the stimulant effect of tea, here is a practical tip: caffeine is very soluble in water; tea polyphenols are not. You can remove most of the caffeine from tea leaves by steeping them in hot water for thirty seconds and draining off the water. Then steep the leaves as you would normally. This will not detract from the flavor or antioxidant activity of what you drink. Try to buy high-quality teas from tea shops, Asian grocery stores, or Internet sites; get organic varieties if you can find them (they are slowly becoming more available in response to consumer demand), and learn to brew them properly.*

By the way, antioxidant polyphenols are also present in

*Two good Web sites are www.inpursuitoftea.com and www.japanese greenteaonline.com.

dark chocolate and in extra-virgin olive oil, foods recommended for inclusion in the diet to promote healthy aging.

Carotenoids are an even larger (more than six hundred now known) family of pigments, even more widely distributed in nature: they occur in algae and some bacteria as well as plants. Animals cannot make them but often put them to use when they eat organisms containing them. The pink coloration in flamingos and salmon is due to carotenoids in their diets, for example. These pigments are fat soluble rather than water soluble. They share a distinctive, common chemical structure, and some are related to vitamin A, an essential micronutrient. Our bodies can make vitamin A from beta-carotene, a principal carotenoid in many fruits and vegetables (mangoes, peaches, carrots, sweet potatoes, spinach), and from a few of its relatives.

Like anthocyanins, the carotenoids interact with light in special ways. This property allows them to help plants photosynthesize as well as protect them from damage by light and oxygen. In humans, they function as biological antioxidants, shielding cells from the destructive effects of free radicals, especially highly reactive, unpaired oxygen atoms. Individual carotenoids may concentrate in particular tissues, offering specific protective effects. For example, lutein, found in collard greens, kale, peas, spinach, and romaine lettuce, is the main carotenoid in the human retina. It reduces the risk of macular degeneration, an age-related disease of the retina that is the commonest cause of loss of vision in the elderly. Lycopene, responsible for the red color of ripe tomatoes, protects the prostate from malignancy. Other carotenoids appear to enhance immune function, protect us from sunburn, and inhibit the development of certain

types of cancer. Again, there is much research on these top-
ics. (An International Symposium on Carotenoids takes
place yearly.)

You want to get as many different kinds of carotenoids
as possible into your diet by eating a great variety of fruits
and vegetables in the red-orange-yellow portion of the
color spectrum. These pigments are more available to the
body from cooked vegetables (carrots, pumpkins, winter
squashes, sweet potatoes, leafy greens) than from raw ones.
And because of their fat solubility, absorption from the gastrointestinal tract is enhanced if fat is present. A marinara
sauce made with olive oil is a great lycopene source, for
example.

The compounds responsible for the attractive colors of
fruits and vegetables represent only some of the phytonutrients that I have called the most important kinds of
micronutrients. Researchers are constantly identifying other
health-protective compounds in plants, like I-3-C in cabbage-
family vegetables and sulforaphane in broccoli, another
cancer fighter. Some phytonutrients are powerful anti-
inflammatory agents. The pungent constituents of ginger
and curcumin in turmeric are good examples, and I urge you
to find ways of consuming more of these culinary spices.
(Remember the turmeric tea that I told you was a popular
cold beverage in Okinawa?) Other phytonutrients modulate
and enhance immune function, maintaining the body's healing system while keeping abnormal inflammation in check.
Still others boost antioxidant defenses to protect DNA and
other cellular components from toxic insults that can cause
direct harm or can promote abnormal inflammation leading
to tissue damage.

The Anti-inflammatory Diet includes as many different plant-derived foods as possible—not only fruits and vegetables but also whole grains, seeds, nuts, herbs, and spices. An active area of nutrition research is even discovering ways that compounds in plants we eat can actually modify the expression of our genes.

10

BODY III: SUPPLEMENTS

Whether or not to use dietary supplements is a contentious issue today. In the recent past, medical authorities told consumers that supplements were a waste of money. Now they say they are dangerous, even life threatening, foisted on a gullible public by an unregulated industry that cares only about profit and is heedless of the harm it causes. On the other side are health experts, including many physicians, who recommend dietary supplements enthusiastically. Some of them are brilliant scientists. Who to believe?

Here are the facts as I see them. I have always stated that supplemental nutrients are not substitutes for the whole foods that contain them. Taking supplements does not excuse you from eating a healthy diet like the one described in the previous chapter (and in Appendix A), with its emphasis on a variety and abundance of fresh fruits and vegetables. This is particularly true for the micronutrients. I take a good daily multivitamin-multimineral supplement, one that I formulated myself, as insurance against gaps in my diet—for example, to cover those days when I am on the road and simply can't get the fruits and vegetables I'd like. The more regularly we supply our bodies with antioxidants and phytonutrients, the better will be our health. Most of us simply can't do that with food, hence the need for supplements. I grow as many vegetables as I can in my winter garden in southern Arizona; I buy organic produce from a local farmer's market, a food co-op, and a healthy supermarket; and I keep my freezer stocked with organic berries. When I am on the road, I do the best I can.

Bear in mind that supplements can only approximate the natural arrays of vitamins, minerals, and protective compounds in plants. For example, nature produces vitamin E in a complex of eight molecules: alpha-, beta-, gamma-, and delta-tocopherols and alpha-, beta-, gamma-, and delta-tocotrienols, all contributing to the antioxidant and protective effects of vitamin-E-containing foods. Most multivitamins provide only alpha-tocopherol, even though research shows the gamma form to be beneficial. Some give you synthetic dl-alpha-tocopherol, half of which is of no use to the human body. Reductionistic researchers conduct clinical studies using only alpha-tocopherol; if the studies are negative, they conclude that vitamin E has no benefit. They haven't tested vitamin E. They have tested only one component of it.

I have told you that there are hundreds of carotenoids with many different protective effects against cancer and other diseases. Most multivitamins give you one: beta-carotene as a precursor of vitamin A. Medical experts used to think that beta-carotene was the most important carotenoid in carrots and other foods that reduce cancer risks. They were wrong. Beta-carotene by itself can actually increase cancer risks in some people (smokers and ex-smokers), because it can act as a pro-oxidant in some circumstances. High-quality multivitamins should give you alpha-carotene as well as the beta form, along with lutein, zeaxanthin, astaxanthin, lycopene, and others. That's better, but it's still not carrots or sweet potatoes. And these products usually give you none of the anthocyanins or representatives of the other classes of plant pigments that make up the rainbow of beneficial phytonutrients.

Apart from providing insurance against gaps in the diet, supplements can provide optimum dosages of natural therapeutic agents that may help prevent and treat age-related diseases. Again, consider vitamin E. Oil-rich seeds and nuts are the main food source of it. Many studies suggest that doses in the range of 200 to 400 IU of alpha-tocopherol (or, better, 80 to 160 milligrams of the whole complex, including tocotrienols) offer the best antioxidant protection against common age-related diseases. Nuts are good for you, but you would have to eat far too many of them to get that amount of vitamin E.

Or look again at indole-3-carbinol (I-3-C), the phytonutrient in cabbage-family vegetables that can reduce breast cancer risk. It does so by influencing estrogen metabolism, probably reducing the risk of other female reproductive system cancers as well. The daily amount of I-3-C that seems to be best for women at high risk for breast cancer is 200 to 400 milligrams a day. They would have to eat a lot of broccoli or kale or brussels sprouts to achieve that level. Not only would that be a chore, it might be hard on some women's digestive systems. Others simply might not like those vegetables. You can easily find 200-milligram capsules of I-3-C in health-food stores and on Internet sites. Critics and foes of the supplement industry say we don't have studies of the safety and efficacy of I-3-C taken in pill form. That's true, and it argues for caution. In my view, the greater concern is safety. Basic toxicity information is available for I-3-C, and I see no cause for alarm with the suggested dosage. I will certainly advise women at high risk for breast cancer to eat their broccoli and brussels sprouts. And I will also make them aware of the alternative of using I-3-C as a dietary supplement.

I should say, too, that I have always favored increased regulation of the dietary supplement industry, which has proved to be incapable of policing itself. Canada has done a better job than the United States in this regard, so that Canadian consumers have access to better products with more informative and accurate labeling. I would like to see the U.S. Food and Drug Administration create a new Division of Natural Therapeutic Agents to regulate herbs, vitamins, minerals, and other products—not with the intent of thwarting consumer access to them but rather of ensuring that products on the market are safe, contain what they claim to contain, and do what they claim to do. It would also be very helpful if physicians, pharmacists, and nurses were knowledgeable about dietary supplements, their benefits and risks, and their possible interactions with prescribed and over-the-counter medications.

You will recall that I said earlier that dietary supplements are a major component of the antiaging medicine that is now so popular. To walk through the exhibit halls at an antiaging medicine convention is to be overwhelmed by people selling pills, capsules, and liquids for claimed life-extending, morbidity-compressing, and age-reversing effects. Most of these are probably not harmful, but most are expensive, and scientific evidence to back up the claims is generally lacking or insufficient for mainstream medical practitioners to feel comfortable with their use.

I wrote at the beginning of this chapter that some brilliant scientists recommend dietary supplements. An example is Bruce Ames, professor of biochemistry and microbiology at the University of California, Berkeley, and a foremost expert on the causation and prevention of cancer. (I have used his publications as a resource on natural toxins in foods.) Recently, he turned his attention to cellular regeneration, in particular to finding ways to slow age-related deterioration of mitochondria. Ames investigated two dietary supplements in rats: alpha-lipoic acid (ALA) and acetyl-L-carnitine (ALCAR). Interest in the former goes back to the 1950s, but ALA was not recognized as an antioxidant until 1988 and was subsequently found to play a central role in energy production within mitochondria. It also appears to decrease insulin resistance and help treat and prevent complications of diabetes, such as peripheral neuropathy. ALCAR, an amino acid derivative, also participates in mitochondrial energy production.

When Ames gave aging rats the two compounds in combination, "they got up and did the Macarena," in his words. "The brain looks better, they are full of energy—everything we looked at looks more like a young animal." The theory behind the treatment is that free radicals, generated by normal metabolism, disable mitochondrial enzymes required for generating energy. The combination of alpha-lipoic acid and acetyl-L-carnitine appears to boost the activity of the enzymes and enable them to burn more fuel.

Ames was so impressed with his results that after publishing them in the *Proceedings of the National Academy of Sciences,* he developed a commercial product, Juvenon, containing the compounds and founded a company to sell it.

In August 2003 the *Berkeley Wellness Letter* reviewed the evidence for the benefits of the components of the product being marketed by one of the university's own faculty members:

Ames and his colleagues have found that high doses of these compounds, in combination, enable elderly rats to function like younger ones. Of course, the same results may not occur in humans. Human studies are just getting started. Though evidence is accumulating, it is clear that the research on ALA is still in its early stages. Large, long-term, well-controlled studies on humans are needed. . . . Though ALA so far appears to be safe, the long-term effects of large supplemental doses are unknown. . . . We still advise waiting until more research has been done.

That is the familiar, conservative voice of mainstream medicine. But how long should we wait? We are all aging, our mitochondria along with everything else. In the absence of medical certainty, what can we do that is likely to be safe and effective to reduce the risks of age-related disease, compress morbidity, and increase the chance of healthy aging? By the time the well-controlled studies on humans are done and analyzed, we might be senescent or dead. Should we take our chances with Juvenon and products like it in the absence of definitive evidence?

You will find my detailed recommendations about dietary supplements in Appendix A. Here I would like to guide you through the major categories of them that I think you should consider adding to your program.

Multivitamins

I recommend taking a daily multivitamin-multimineral product that meets the following specifications:

- It should not contain any preformed vitamin A (retinol).
- It should give you a mixture of carotenoids, not just beta-carotene. This should include lutein and lycopene, as well as other members of this family of antioxidant pigments.
- It should provide vitamin E as mixed, natural tocopherols, not just as d-alpha-tocopherol or, worse, synthetic dl-alpha-tocopherol. Better-quality products will also provide mixed tocotrienols, the other components of the natural vitamin E complex.
- It should provide 50 milligrams each of most B vitamins, except for folic acid (at least 400 micrograms) and vitamin B_{12} (at least 50 micrograms).
- It need not contain much more than 200 milligrams of vitamin C, which is all the human body can use in a day.
- It should provide at least 400 IU of vitamin D, but note that you will need to take additional vitamin D to get to my recommended daily intake of 1,000 IU.
- It should not contain iron, unless you are a menstruating woman, are pregnant, or have documented iron-deficiency anemia.
- It should have no more than 200 micrograms of selenium, a key antioxidant mineral.
- It should provide some calcium, preferably as calcium citrate, although most women will need to take additional calcium to maintain bone health.

Such a product will probably require taking more than one pill or capsule. You can take it any time of day, but always do so with a full stomach to avoid indigestion. Vitamins D and E and the carotenoids need fat to be absorbed. Do not take them with, for example, a low-fat breakfast such as a half grapefruit, a bowl of oatmeal, and tea or coffee.

Most women should take 500 to 700 milligrams of calcium as a supplement, preferably as calcium citrate taken with meals for best absorption. Men should get no more than 700 milligrams daily from all sources and do not need to supplement.

Additional Antioxidant Support

In addition to the antioxidants you get from eating fruits and vegetables, from tea, dark chocolate, and olive oil, and from your multivitamin-multimineral supplement (vitamin C, carotenoids, vitamin E, and selenium), you might consider a few natural products that provide additional antioxidant support. Remember, this is a tricky area, where scientific evidence is deficient and theoretical concerns exist about a possible downside of taking antioxidants in supplement form (see pages 97–102). Nevertheless, most of the supplements recommended by practitioners of antiaging medicine are antioxidants. I would consider taking only those with the most supporting science behind them:

- *Co-Q-10* (coenzyme Q, or ubiquinone) is made naturally in the body. In addition to acting as an antioxidant, it increases oxygen use at the cellular level, improving the function of heart muscle cells and boosting capacity for aerobic exercise. It is much researched and widely used. I take it myself, frequently recommend it to patients, including those with cancer, diabetes, and gum disease, and think its benefits outweigh any risks. The main problem with it is bioavailability—how much gets into the system and gets used. New softgel and emulsified forms are much better absorbed but still must be taken with a fat-containing meal. I recommend 60 milligrams a day of one of the new forms. Note that the widely prescribed statin drugs inhibit the body's own production of this compound; anyone on a statin should be taking supplemental Co-Q-10.

- *Grape seed extract* and *pine bark extract* are sources of a group of flavonoids called proanthocyanidins, or PCOs, related to the red and purple anthocyanin pigments discussed earlier. Many practitioners recommend these supplements for the prevention and treatment of particular age-related diseases, including cardiovascular disease, cataracts, and macular degeneration. In the absence of specific ailments, they suggest a daily dose of 100 milligrams to maintain general health. An extract of the bark of the French maritime pine, sold under the brand name Pycnogenol, is equivalent, in my opinion, to cheaper grape seed extract. I do not take either of these, because my diet is rich in flavonoids from tea, berries and other fruits, vegetables, and dark chocolate, and I already take plenty of supplements. But you might consider these products for additional antioxidant support if you are not consuming enough dietary sources of flavonoids.

- *Alpha-lipoic acid* (with or without acetyl-L-carnitine) is interesting to me because it decreases insulin resistance while augmenting the body's antioxidant defenses. If you have any degree of metabolic syndrome (low HDL cholesterol, high serum triglycerides, a tendency to gain weight in the abdomen, a tendency toward high blood pressure) or have a personal or family history of obesity or type 2 diabetes, it might be worth taking ALA as a supplemental antioxidant. Start with 100 milligrams a day; you can take up to 400 milligrams a day.

Anti-inflammatory Support

In addition to eating an anti-inflammatory diet, you might want to give your body additional support with supplements. Some culinary herbs have powerful anti-inflammatory effects. There are also familiar over-the-counter drugs.

- *Ginger and turmeric.* Of course, you can add these closely related spices to food, easier in the case of the former, unless you cook a lot of Indian food. People in our culture like ginger tea and ginger candies (have you ever had dark-chocolate-coated slices of candied ginger? Try them) and are happy to flavor cakes and cookies with this spice, but they are unlikely to get enough of it regularly to affect inflammation. Dried ginger is a more powerful anti-inflammatory agent than fresh, because there is a chemical conversion of constituents on drying that favor this effect. Capsules of dried, powdered ginger are sold in health-food stores; some are standardized for content of active components. The recommended starting dose is 1 gram a day (usually 2 capsules), taken after a meal to avoid stomach irritation. I know a number of people whose musculoskeletal and other ailments disappeared after using ginger in this way for several months. There is no reason not to stay on it indefinitely.

  Turmeric is more of a problem, because it has a bitter taste in large amounts, and it can stain teeth and clothing bright yellow. Americans know it as the principal ingredient in the mild yellow prepared mustard they like and in occasional exotic curries. Otherwise, they would have no idea how to get enough of it in food to affect inflammatory status. I am working to make the instant turmeric tea of Okinawa available here, in part because I would like to drink it myself. As with ginger, you can find turmeric products in health-food stores, but most are preparations of curcumin, which is only one of the active components. I suggest you take a whole extract of turmeric, such as one prepared by the process of "supercritical extraction," which uses liquefied carbon dioxide as a solvent.

Turmeric may have a specific preventive effect against Alzheimer's disease. The population of rural India has one of the lowest rates of this disease in the world; daily consumption of turmeric may be a factor, because animal experiments with it demonstrate a protective effect. I believe it reduces the risk of cancer as well.

You might want to look for products that combine extracts of ginger and turmeric in the same capsule, adding other anti-inflammatory herbs such as rosemary, green tea, and holy basil *(Ocimum sanctum)* from India. I have used these combination products successfully to treat both minor and major inflammatory disorders, enabling patients to reduce dosages of standard anti-inflammatory drugs or eliminate them completely. (See Appendix B for details.)

- *Aspirin* offers a great many health benefits, including downregulation of inflammation. Its reduction of heart attack risk may derive from that property but is usually thought to be due to its action on platelets. It makes them less sticky, less likely to clump together and initiate blood clots, which are the immediate causes of coronary occlusions. This blood-thinning effect is a consequence of its influence on the same hormones that mediate inflammation. And, as I explained in the previous chapter, there is an accompanying reduction of cancer risk as well, because those hormones also increase cell proliferation and the risk of malignant transformation. The best evidence here is for prevention of colorectal cancer, one of the major killing cancers in the West. Aspirin may also reduce the risk of cancer of the esophagus and some other organs.

There is a downside to aspirin, mainly irritation and bleeding of the lining of the stomach and lower GI tract. (It can also initiate asthma attacks in some susceptible individuals and slightly increases the risk of hemorrhagic strokes, which are rare events to begin with.) In general, the health benefits of low-dose aspirin regimens greatly outweigh the risks. I take two baby aspirins a day (81 milligrams each or 162 milligrams total), equivalent to half of an adult tablet.

- *Other NSAIDs* (nonsteroidal anti-inflammatory drugs), aside from aspirin, include ibuprofen (sold as Motrin and Advil) and related products. Ibuprofen reduces the risk of Alzheimer's disease more than aspirin and has the same risks of gastrointestinal irritation and bleeding. I would recommend it for daily use only to those with symptomatic inflammation (like arthritis or bursitis) or a significant family history of Alzheimer's.

Body Composition Support

The hormone DHEA (dehydroepiandrosterone), made in the adrenal gland and available in synthetic form as a supplement, shows promise in reversing some of the changes in body composition that accompany aging. It increases bone density and skin thickness and tone, and also decreases abdominal fat in elderly men and women. Abdominal fat is more of a health risk than fat elsewhere in the body because it is associated with metabolic syndrome and increased risk of heart attack and stroke. The decrease in abdominal fat promoted by DHEA also results in an increase in insulin sensitivity. Finally, this hormone can improve erectile dysfunction in men and increase libido in both men and women.

DHEA is the precursor of both male and female sex hormones. Natural production peaks at about twenty to thirty years of age and then declines steadily. Its supplemental use during routine aging is not yet endorsed by mainstream medical doctors, who want to see more and larger studies of it, but antiaging doctors routinely prescribe it and say they see few adverse effects. Some masculinizing changes (acne, hair loss, excessive hair growth, and deepening of the voice) have been reported in women. DHEA may slightly increase risks of breast and prostate cancer, affect liver function and blood pressure, and alter metabolism of prescribed medications.

The recommended dose of DHEA in routine aging is 25–50 milligrams a day. It may take six months of use to see desired effects. I consider this hormone to be relatively safe and effective, but I do not recommend trying it without first discussing the benefits and risks with your physician.

Immune Support

Our immune systems weaken as we age, making us more susceptible to infections and cancer and slowing our healing responses. In addition, the immune systems of both old and young are under constant assault from toxins in the environment, both natural and man-made. Living in crowded cities, traveling frequently in airplanes, and spending time in day care centers and schools all expose us to many more germs than people had to deal with in the past. We can protect and strengthen our immunity by eating right, getting enough activity and rest, practicing stress reduction, and cultivating healthy emotional states. It is also worth knowing about and experimenting with natural products that enhance immune function.

We don't have a good name for this class of remedies, usually called tonics or adaptogens. The former term sounds distinctly unscientific, conjuring up images of nostrums sold out of medicine wagons in an earlier age. The latter, coined by Soviet scientists in the mid–twentieth century, is cumbersome, with an unclear meaning. Whatever you call them, these herbs and mushrooms are most useful. They are non-toxic, can be used for extended periods, and definitely work. I wrote about reishi and arctic root *(Rhodiola)* earlier (see page 50). Here I will mention two immune-enhancing products that I use myself and recommend frequently:

- *Astragalus,* obtained from the root of *Astragalus membranaceus* in the pea family, has a long history in Chinese medicine, where it is used to ward off colds and flu. Chinese people cook slices of the pleasant-tasting dried root in chicken and duck broth to make a tonic soup, and extracts are sold in all Chinese pharmacies under the name *hoangqi.* Research confirms the antiviral and immune-enhancing properties of the root. It is plentiful and inexpensive.

  I often recommend it to people who "get everything going around," to cancer patients undergoing chemo-therapy that suppresses the bone marrow, to those with immune deficiencies, and to healthy people through the entirety of the flu season. Look for standardized extracts in capsules and take the daily dosage given on the label.

- *Immune-enhancing mushrooms* include edible species like shiitake, maitake, and oyster mushrooms as well as purely medicinal ones like reishi that are too bitter and woody to be used as food. All are nontoxic and can be used indefinitely as dietary supplements. Research on these mushrooms is extensive, including identification of active compounds, a great many animal studies, and more and more clinical investigations in cases of infectious disease, cancer, and AIDS. Long valued in the traditional medicines of China, Korea, and Japan, these mushrooms are now attracting more interest from researchers and clinicians in the West.

I believe it is better to take a number of these mushrooms together, because their effects are synergistic. Liquid, powder, and encapsulated forms are available, some providing extracts of seven or more species. The product I take every day contains a dozen different ones, with such exotic names as *agarikon, zhu ling, yun zhi, chaga,* and *himematsutake.* It is a liquid extract, whose taste is not disagreeable. I take a dropperful of it in a little water twice a day and believe it makes me resistant to germs and better able to handle periods of intensive travel and attendance at public events. (I also add a spoonful of a dry version of the same product to my dogs' food once a day to reduce their risk of cancer, which has become ever more frequent in canines.) You will find details about where to find these products in Appendix B.

Detoxification

Protection from toxins begins with minimizing exposure to them, as by not smoking, by drinking purified water, by eating pesticide-free food as often as possible, by eating lower on the food chain, by not ingesting toxic substances, and by not living near hazardous sites like toxic-waste dumps. You can help the body rid itself of toxins by drinking plenty of pure water, having regular bowel movements, breathing clean air deeply, and sweating. This last technique is particularly effective, and I recommend that you find ways to sit in saunas or steam baths as often as you can, making sure that you drink enough water when you do.

Because the main organ responsible for processing toxins is the liver, it is worth knowing about an herbal remedy with an excellent reputation for protecting and enhancing liver function. It is milk thistle, an extract of the seeds of a common European plant *(Silybum marianum)*, now naturalized in North America. Milk thistle is nontoxic and can be used for extended periods. Anyone who drinks alcohol heavily, who takes drugs or medications that can harm the liver, who has abnormal liver function for any reason, or who works with solvents or has a history of toxic exposures should take milk thistle. Look for extracts standardized to 70 to 80 percent silymarin, the active fraction, and take two capsules twice a day or as the label directs.

Energy Support

A common complaint of older people is waning energy. This is probably the main indication for tonic herbs and mushrooms. I will list my favorites and describe their particular benefits, but you will have to experiment with them to find out which ones work best for you. I suggest choosing and trying each one daily for two months. Then assess its value. If you like its effects, you can stay on these herbs indefinitely, perhaps giving yourself occasional breaks—say, two or three weeks off every four months or so.

- *Ginseng.* Asian ginseng *(Panax ginseng)* and American ginseng *(Panax quinquefolius)* are both in great demand worldwide. The Asian species is more of a stimulant and more esteemed as a sexual energizer for men. American ginseng is valued for its adaptogenic (stress-protective) properties. Chinese ginseng connoisseurs warn not to waste this root in your youth; save it for old age, they say, then see what it can do for you. Buy only extracts that are standardized for ginsenoside content, follow dosage recommendations on labels, and do not expect to notice results until after six to eight weeks of regular use.
- *Eleuthero ginseng,* formerly called Siberian ginseng, comes from a plant *(Eleutherococcus senticosus)* that is related to true ginseng. It has a long history of use by athletes, military personnel, and cosmonauts of the former Soviet Union and is also in great demand. Buy only products that are standardized for eleutheroside content and follow dosage recommendations on labels, also waiting six to eight weeks to evaluate the effect.
- *Arctic root,* or *Rhodiola,* is the plant I discussed earlier as a possible antiaging remedy. It does not have that property but does enhance endurance, reduce harmful effects of stress, and improve mood and memory. Some people report increased sexual energy from it as well. Rhodiola seems to work faster than ginseng or eleuthero, possibly

in just two weeks. Look for products standardized to 3 percent rosavins and 1 percent salidroside, and follow dosage recommendations on labels.

- *Cordyceps* is a mushroom from China, much used in that country as an energizing tonic for people debilitated by age, illness, or injury. It is also used by athletes to increase aerobic capacity and endurance. Wild cordyceps parasitizes the larvae of certain moths; the preparation used in China is the whole, dried mushroom attached to a mummified larva, simmered in soup. Here you can get extracts of cordyceps cultivated on grain in either liquid or capsule form.

Sexual Support

Declining sexual interest and energy are common complaints of older people, and, as you might expect, many products are offered for sale to improve them, including prescription drugs like Viagra, herbs like ginseng, and dietary supplements like the amino acid L-arginine. Before I review them, I should point out that some thoughtful persons have welcomed the sexual decline of old age instead of desperately seeking remedies for it. For example, in a famous essay, "On Old Age," the Roman orator, politician, and philosopher Marcus Tullius Cicero (106–43 B.C.E.) wrote: "Now we come to [another] accusation people make against old age: sex—or rather, the absence of it. But in fact it is a great compensation of age that it frees us from what is the source of so much corruption when we are younger." Cicero goes on to elaborate the ways in which desire for sexual gratification can dominate the mind and interfere with the pursuit of excellence in life. He would not be a good spokesperson for

Viagra. I realize that his view is not popular today, but I would like you to consider it.

Here is a quick review of natural remedies for age-related sexual deficiency:

- *Testosterone,* the male hormone, can in low doses give a remarkable boost to postmenopausal women experiencing lack of interest in sex. It is a prescription drug that comes in pill or topical forms and should not be used unless blood tests reveal a deficiency. (Women produce testosterone naturally, though in much smaller amounts than men, and it exerts a strong influence on female libido.) Men with demonstrated testosterone deficiency will also benefit, but men who take more testosterone than they need are likely to become more aggressive rather than more sexual. The hormone can also increase their risks of atherosclerosis and prostate disease. Like all hormones, testosterone should be used only under medical supervision.
- *Asian ginseng* (see page 213) is probably the most widely used herbal sex enhancer for men.
- *Ashwagandha* is an herb from India *(Withania somnifera)* much used in Ayurvedic medicine and sometimes called "Indian ginseng," although it is unrelated to true ginseng. It is much more available and consequently much less expensive than ginseng, and, unlike ginseng, it has a calming, mildly sedative action rather than a stimulating one. Indians value it as a sexual enhancer, again mainly for men, and as a general tonic and adaptogen. Look for extracts standardized to 1.5 percent withanolides and 1 percent alkaloids. Give it a six-to-eight-week trial.
- *Rhodiola* (see above, pages 50 and 213).

These are the main categories of supplements I would consider as part of a program for healthy aging. You will, of course, hear and read about many other products, especially from the antiaging crowd. *Caveat emptor*—buyer beware!

11

BODY IV: PHYSICAL ACTIVITY

It is probably possible to lead an inactive life and still experience healthy aging, but it isn't likely. Maintenance of physical activity throughout life and successful aging go hand in hand; this was one of the strongest correlations found in the MacArthur Foundation's Study of Aging in America, as reported in 1998 in the book *Successful Aging*. Almost all of the healthy seniors I know were physically active throughout life, and many of them still are. They walk, dance, play golf, swim, lift weights, do yoga and tai chi. Some of them are more engaged in physical activity than their middle-aged counterparts.

In Japan, which still boasts the world's highest longevity at an average of almost eighty years, not only are numbers of centenarians increasing but so are the numbers of "super seniors," extraordinarily fit oldsters. Here is a description of one:

> As dawn breaks over the world's largest metropolis, Keizo Miura, a sinewy centenarian, is already dressed in his charcoal gray tracksuit and pumped to sweat.
>
> Before a hearty breakfast of seaweed and eggs, Miura races through his indoor exercises, wincing as

his neck—still tender from a collarbone injury—momentarily reminds him that he was born in 1904. The man who has become a role model in graying Japan sucks it up, shaking off the pain the way he did last year when he skied down Europe's Mont Blanc at age ninety-nine. In a Tokyo minute, he is out the front door for his daily two-mile power walk.

"I still feel good," said Miura, who in 1981 became the oldest man to scale Mount Kilimanjaro, Africa's tallest peak, and is training for an expedition to the Italian Alps next year. "There's really nothing so amazing about me . . . but my son, now he is amazing."

That would be Yuichiro Miura, seventy-two, who in May 2003 became the oldest man to reach the summit of Mount Everest.

I could fill this chapter with accounts of old people who are setting records and astounding the rest of us with their physical achievements, people in their eighties and nineties still pumping iron, surfing, competing in triathlons, and otherwise showing us that the human body can keep it up in ways our parents and grandparents might not have been able to imagine. As friends and acquaintances learned that I was writing on healthy aging, they invited me to meet American super seniors and watch them doing power yoga, dance marathons, and other extraordinary feats.

All of this is inspiring and of special interest to antiaging enthusiasts, but it is peripheral to what I have to tell you in this chapter. I am concerned with ordinary life and with what all of us need to know about physical activity and aging, even if we are not planning to climb mountains—*especially* if we are not planning to climb mountains. In traditional cultures, it is the activities of daily living that condition the physical body. For example, the healthy old people I met in Okinawa had not run marathons; they worked the soil by hand, chopped wood, carried water, went into the mountains to gather wild vegetables, cast fishing nets, and walked and walked all their lives.

The human body is designed for this kind of regular and varied use. Modern life often foils that purpose, forcing too many of us to spend most of our days sitting at desks and getting around in cars. We have to get our physical activity by taking periods of exercise, which is often not varied. This is regrettable, but it is as it is. Given the limitations of modern life, how can we fulfill the body's requirement for the physical activity it needs in order to age gracefully? To do so, you need to understand both the benefits and the risks of physical activity.

I will write about the risks first, because I rarely hear them explained clearly and exercise enthusiasts do not like to acknowledge them, much less discuss them.

Let me start by saying it is possible to get too much physical activity, not just because overactivity raises the possibility of damaging joints, muscles, and bones but also because of possible adverse effects on body composition, the nervous system, and reproductive and immune function. As to the former, I will simply note that doctors who care for people who have done physical labor all their lives know how high is the incidence of degenerative joint disease, repetitive strain injury, and other musculoskeletal calamities in this group. These problems often greatly restrict physical activity in old age and detract from quality of life. They may be less common in traditional cultures, like that of rural Okinawa in the past century, because physical activity there was so varied. Workers in our society are more likely to do the same physical activity over and over, putting them at risk for injury. And let me remind young readers that injuries from contact sports often result in musculoskeletal and neurological problems that will plague you when you are older by limiting your mobility. Knees are especially vulnerable, and surgical methods for repairing them are less than ideal. Repeated concussive injuries, as in football and soccer, may be associated with cognitive impairment in later life. Choose your sports carefully.

Young female athletes stop menstruating if they are too active because their body fat drops below the level that their reproductive systems regard as safe for conception; without adequate caloric reserves a pregnancy cannot be carried to term. This change in body composition may have other, less apparent consequences for long-term health. In particular, it may expose the nervous and immune systems to potential harm from environmental toxins.

The central nervous system is fatty tissue, built of special kinds of lipids. Many pesticides and environmental toxins are fat soluble. If you are exposed to them and have little body fat to dilute them, they are likely to concentrate in nervous tissue, where they can initiate destructive processes that lead to neurodegenerative disease. Perhaps this is the reason that ALS (amyotrophic lateral sclerosis) appears more frequently in athletes. At the Integrative Medicine Clinic at the University of Arizona, I have seen a number of men in their thirties with this devastating diagnosis, an unusually young age group for the onset of ALS. All had a history of participating in extreme sports and competitive, ultra-athletic events, and all were extraordinarily lean.

Many people assume that ultra-athletes must be ultra-healthy and that the less body fat you have the better off you are in terms of health and longevity. That may not be the case. It is possible that intense physical activity and extreme leanness do correlate with better cardiovascular health and very low risk of type 2 diabetes, but there may be a trade-off in terms of neurological health. In addition, those with very little body fat are at higher risk of death from acute infectious disease, which often places extreme metabolic demands on the body. Severe febrile illnesses like influenza and pneumonia cause rapid loss of weight—ten pounds or more in a few days. If you have no weight to spare, your odds of surviving this kind of crisis are lower than those of your heftier fellows.

There is another danger of excessive physical activity, one that should be obvious but is never mentioned. You will recall that normal metabolism is the most significant source of oxidative stress and that the body's antioxidant defenses have evolved to contain it. When you rev up your metabolism, as in periods of aerobic exercise, you increase oxidative stress. Aerobic exercise is a powerful generator of free radicals. Too much of it can overwhelm our defenses, leaving bodies more susceptible over time to age-related diseases. Maybe this is another reason for seeing the early onset of rare neurodegenerative disease in relatively young extreme athletes.

I present these ideas in order to argue for moderation in exercise (as in other things), not to help you justify being overweight or sedentary. Far more people in our culture err on the side of getting too little physical activity than too much. Just be aware that too much physical activity or the wrong kind of physical activity can directly damage the structure of the body, leave it more vulnerable to toxins and other agents of disease, and overtax its defenses against oxidative stress. In addition to figuring out how much activity you need to give your body to help it age well, you must be informed about the kinds of activity that serve it best.

Under the heading of "physical activity," I include the following components, each of which serves quite different purposes, although all are necessary for optimum health as you age.

Aerobic exercise ("cardio") is any activity that increases heart rate and makes you huff and puff. In light stages of it, you can carry on a normal conversation. In moderate stages, talking becomes difficult, and in intense stages, you breathe very hard and cannot talk. Cardiovascular fitness is indicated by the ability to meet aerobic challenges such as running fast for short distances and climbing flights of stairs as well as by quick recovery, with heart rate dropping back to normal within a few minutes of the cessation of work. This sort of activity, especially sustained moderate forms, perhaps with some of the high-intensity sort, is necessary to maintain the cardiovascular system in good condition. It tones the heart muscle, improves the elasticity of arteries, helps counteract the age-related rise in blood pressure so common in our population, and develops collateral circulation in the heart, protecting it against possible obstructions in coronary artery flow. It also tunes metabolism, maintaining sensitivity of cells to insulin and opposing the development of metabolic syndromes that lead to obesity.

In addition, aerobic exercise burns calories and is the best way to prevent weight gain if you are consuming more calories than your body needs. Exercise by itself rarely corrects obesity unless it is accompanied by a change in eating habits, but it can prevent it, and, as I noted previously, for those who cannot get their weight down to recommended levels, regular aerobic exercise is absolutely necessary to maintain optimum health.

Aerobic exercise has so many benefits on physiology that I do not have space to list them all. I will mention that it improves immune function and cognitive function and has a marked effect on mood. By increasing production of endorphins, the body's own molecules that behave like opiates, it both treats and prevents depression without the side effects of antidepressant drugs. By the way, this last effect accounts for the potential addictiveness of aerobic exercise. Like any addiction, compulsive exercising limits your freedom and wastes energy; it can also expose you to the risks of excessive physical activity that I have discussed. I do not recommend it.

It is desirable, though, to engage in aerobic activity every day—that is, to do something that gets you into the zone of hard breathing and increased heart rate. You don't have to work out in a gym to accomplish that. You can do it by walking, climbing stairs, doing house- and yard work, and any number of other ordinary tasks. It's better if you can sustain moderate aerobic activity for thirty minutes or more, but if you have to get it in bits and pieces throughout the day, that's fine too.

As you get older, you will want to select your aerobic activities with care, making sure they are suited to your body and not likely to lead to injury. For example, running is generally more appropriate for younger folks. It can be aerobically intense, is great for burning calories, and can deliver a terrific endorphin high, but unless you are thin and light boned, it can easily damage your joints. I see far too many middle-aged men who "ran through the pain," ignoring protests from their bodies, and now are limited in what they can do physically as a result.

Let me describe the kinds of aerobic activity I like and make part of my routine:

- *Walking* is the overall best exercise that can fulfill the body's need for regular aerobic activity, if you do it vigorously enough. I have long promoted walking as an excellent form of exercise because it requires no equipment, everyone knows how to do it, and it carries the lowest risk of injury. The human body is designed to walk. You can walk in parks or shopping malls or in front of your house. I love to walk around my desert property, going up and down hills and along creek beds. When I am away from home, I always try to walk every day, but I am dismayed by how unfriendly to walkers most cities in North America are, with the exception of New York. Manhattan is the only American city in which people walk everywhere, much as they do in all cities in Japan. Japanese walk a lot, they walk fast, and they are constantly going up and down flights of steps to catch commuter trains and subways. Manhattan is also the only American city where the great American obesity epidemic is not so visible, and there is no doubt in my mind that a cause-and-effect relationship with walking exists.

  To get maximum benefit from walking, aim for forty-five minutes a day, an average of five days a week. Include some stretches of uphill and fast walking to get your heart and respiratory rates into the zone where talking becomes a bit difficult. Get good walking shoes from a store that specializes in sports footwear and replace them when they wear out. You can also join walking clubs, learn power walking, go on walking tours in Europe, use walking poles (something like ski poles; see Appendix B for a source) to assist you on uneven ground, walk with friends and dogs. Just do it. Also, practice parking farther away rather than closer to destinations when you drive in order to balance sedentary time in the car.

And please use stairs when possible. I often walk up seven flights at the University of Arizona Health Sciences Center on days when I am in the Integrative Medicine Clinic and unable to get other aerobic activity. When I do take an elevator, I am usually accompanied by people who ride up two floors or even one. (Many of them are overweight and returning from the cafeteria with a soft drink in one hand and a pastry or carton of fries in the other. Do we need to look further for causes of obesity in our country?)

Walking is a perfect conditioner for joints. It can take you to interesting places and can serve you your whole life. Even if you are very old and have little energy for the aerobic activities of youth, you can walk around your house.

- *Swimming.* I love to swim. It requires that I use my body in a different way from other forms of exercise, forces me to breathe consciously and efficiently, is great for my muscles and joints, and provides a pleasant altered state of consciousness that helps me dissipate tension—a welcome break from desk work. But I can't tolerate most swimming pools because of their chlorine, which I find very irritating. I have a wonderful aboveground pool at my home that I disinfect with a copper-silver ion generator, much superior to a chlorine system. (I can swim underwater in it with my eyes open with no discomfort.) Other nonchlorine technologies exist as well (see Appendix B). The obstacles to greater use of them in public pools is the resistance of pool maintenance companies, which do not understand them, and obsolete health-department regulations in some places.

At home, I swim laps for twenty to thirty minutes most

days, unless the weather is very bad. (The pool is heated, by the sun most of the year.) In the summers, when I am at my northern retreat in Canada, there is a lake that I try to swim in every day. It's colder than my pool but so clean that you can drink the water as you swim in it. And there's an island in the middle of it that makes for an aerobic challenge. I start out with a crawl, switching to backstroke and breaststroke when my crawling muscles get fatigued.

Swimming is great for older people whose joints are troublesome. Many spas and retirement communities offer group classes in water aerobics or "aquacise" that are most enjoyable. Find out where you can join them.

Here are two tips on swimming that you might not know. Try using fins to increase the power of your kicking; they make a great difference. Also consider swimming with a mask and snorkel, which will allow you to move through the water without turning and raising your head to breathe. Most people turn their heads in only one direction when they swim, straining their neck muscles in the process.

- *Cycling.* I have a mountain bike with front and rear shock absorbers, easy gears, and a comfortable seat. I ride it on the dirt roads around my property and into the adjacent national park. I do not have to deal with cars or their exhaust fumes. I get to see beautiful scenery. And I go up some long hills that are definitely aerobic work. Coming back downhill is lots of fun. I ride my bike a couple of times a week, more in the spring and fall, when the days are just right. In Canada, I can get around a lot by bike. Cycling provides a good workout for my leg muscles and my heart and lungs, and I find it to be a perfect complement to swimming.

I see many older people riding bikes on paved roads outside of Tucson, many in recumbent bikes or on tandem bikes. Please be aware of the hazards of cycling, which mainly have to do with cars. Make sure you have a bike that fits you properly, wear a helmet, and make use of all safety measures to reduce risk of accidents. Always pay attention if you are on heavily traveled roads.

- *Exercise machines* are convenient for indoor activity. You can use them at gyms or get one for your home. I like the elliptical trainer, because it is easy on the knees and adds arm motion to the usual striding. On days when I don't or can't swim or walk outside, I try to do a thirty-minute session of cardio on this machine, usually following an interval program that takes resistance up for one to three minutes, putting me in the moderate-to-intense zone with recovery in between. I work up a good sweat in a half hour. In gyms, I might use a stationary bike or stair climber if an elliptical trainer is not available, and occasionally a treadmill. I have to say, however, that I find all of these boring, especially treadmills, and need to find ways to distract myself to make the experience more interesting. I have my home elliptical trainer in a room with a television and often watch movies as I exercise. Sometimes, I put on a headset and listen to an audiobook. Both strategies work well for me.

I strongly recommend getting a piece of exercise equipment for your home, but be sure you are committed to using it. I see too many aerobic machines gathering dust in garages or used as clothes racks in bedrooms. Also, investigate the options thoroughly before you buy, making sure the equipment is right for you and your budget. If you can get an exercise machine for a free trial period, do so. Try also to get a salesperson or trainer to watch you on it to make sure you are in the right position and using it correctly.

All of these forms of aerobic exercise are appropriate for people of all ages.

To repeat and summarize what I have written in this section: Regular aerobic exercise is a requirement for healthy aging. Ideally, you should get some every day, and it should be varied to maximize benefits and minimize risks. I advise you at the outset to aim for an average of thirty minutes of some sustained aerobic activity an average of five days a week. Go for moderate intensity: hard breathing, some interference with talking. In the case of walking, which I recommend highly, make it forty-five minutes if possible. In addition, try to make ordinary activities like housework and shopping more aerobic by moving faster.

Strength training is the second component of physical activity that your body needs. Its purpose is to build and maintain bone and muscle mass, both of which diminish with age as a result of changes in hormone levels and metabolism. Loss of bone mineral density leads to osteopenia, then to osteoporosis, which predisposes one to fractures and disability in later life. To avoid those problems, you need to build up sufficient bone mass early in life, especially in adolescence and young adulthood. (Maximum bone mass is reached around age thirty-five.) You then have to lead a lifestyle that maintains rather than lessens it. This is especially important for females, because declining levels of sex hormones after menopause put them at risk much earlier in life than men. To build bone mass when young, you have to eat right (plenty of green vegetables, sources of calcium, and vitamin D), get adequate physical activity, and avoid behaviors that promote loss of bone density, such as smoking and consuming large amounts of soda, coffee, alcohol, and sugar. To preserve bone mass in midlife and old age, you must give your body strength training, sometimes called resistance exercise.

Bone is constantly being re-formed by the action of opposing forces, some destructive, some constructive, in response to the stresses and demands placed on it. These changes are under precise cellular and hormonal control and can take place very quickly. Resistance exercise places demands on bone that cause the constructive influences to dominate, halting loss of mineral density and even adding to it.

Everyone does some of this sort of work as part of daily routines, whenever we lift, pull, or push something heavy, for example. Some of the aerobic activities described above, like walking and climbing stairs, build strength, but others do not. In swimming, the force of gravity is neutralized by the buoyancy of water, and in cycling, whether on a regular bike or a stationary one, the bicycle frame carries most of your weight. The best way to maintain bone density is by doing weight training, with either resistance machines or free weights.

This will also build and maintain muscle mass, equally important as you age. In addition to protecting and stabilizing joints and giving you the strength you need to enjoy life, good muscle mass optimizes metabolism and protects from obesity and its complications. The reason is that muscle, unlike fat, is a metabolic furnace. The more muscle you have, the more calories you can burn and the less likely you are to develop insulin resistance. As in the case of bone, muscle mass is easily added in early life, when hormone levels are high and metabolism is active. For this reason, I often encourage the interest that many teenagers have in body-building.

I note, however, that most bodybuilders are into it for the sake of appearance, men especially, who easily get obsessed with "bulking up." This focus often leads them to ingest excessive amounts of protein, take dietary supplements supposed to increase muscle mass, and experiment with anabolic steroids in addition to working out compulsively, all of which may undermine long-term health. Such behavior in men seems analogous to eating disorders in women obsessed with being thin; in fact, similar neurochemical disturbances may link the two. In my view, the cosmetic effects of strength training are incidental to its true value in maintaining healthy bone and muscle mass into old age.

Bodybuilders are often dismayed at how quickly their hard-earned buffed appearance fades if they stop their weight-lifting routines. One competitive bodybuilder told me he had "deflated like a balloon" when he quit. But this quick responsiveness of muscles to work is equal cause for happiness: you will see the results of starting strength training very quickly. Bones respond just as fast, but we cannot sense our bone density the way we can see and feel the mass and tone of our muscles.

You can start strength training and get benefit from it at any age. It can even improve the physical and mental well-being of old people in assisted-living facilities. If you have not done this sort of activity before, however, I would urge you to start slowly and begin by working with an expert, a personal trainer or an instructor in a gym. It is most important to use resistance equipment correctly, both to minimize risks and maximize benefits. Do not invest in any equipment for the home without researching it thoroughly. There are many options, ranging from expensive machines and elaborate arrays of free weights to very inexpensive and highly portable sets of rubber tubing—lengths in various thicknesses with handles on the ends that are most efficient once you learn how to use them. They can be used to work all the major muscle groups.

In general, you will want to do strength training two to three days a week, allowing recovery days in between the sessions. Doing it more frequently will be counterproductive. You should be able to learn a routine, whether with machines, free weights, or tubing, that you can complete in half an hour.

One form of strength training that has become fashionable of late is the Pilates method, invented by Joseph Pilates and developed further by his wife, Clara, in the early part of the last century. Long popular with dancers, it is now in vogue with fitness-conscious people of all ages and backgrounds. The Pilates system uses special machines and is usually taught in studios or fitness clubs by trained instructors. It emphasizes correct posture and makes use of stretching as well as working muscles against resistance. It also uses spring tension, straps to hold feet or hands, and supports for the back, neck, and shoulders. Group classes done on mats may cost $20 an hour, while one-on-one instruction using all the Pilates equipment may cost $100 an hour. You will find Pilates instructors and studios in most cities. The people I know who use this method are enthusiastic about it, but remember, you can work your muscles at home with rubber tubing for next to nothing.

Flexibility and balance training is the final component of physical activity I want you to know about. Its purpose is to reduce the kinds of physical discomfort that bother older people as well as to protect you from falls. Falls are a major cause of disability and worse in the elderly. You can protect yourself in two ways: by addressing potential hazards in your environment and by attending to your body's capacity to compensate quickly for sudden twists, bumps, and skids.

Aches and pains are high on the list of complaints of old age. Many of them are avoidable, the result of chronic muscle tension and stiffness of joints that simple flexibility training can prevent by toning muscles and keeping joints lubricated. You do some of this whenever you stretch. Watch dogs and cats do it to get an idea of how natural it is to stretch. The general principle is simple: whenever the body has been in one position for a while, it is good to stretch it in an opposite position briefly. For example, if you spend time working at a desktop computer, get up periodically and extend the back and neck by arching them backward.

The best-known formal system of stretching is yoga, now immensely popular in the West. A philosophy and practice intended to facilitate union with higher consciousness, yoga includes dietary principles, hygienic techniques, breathing exercises, meditations, and postures (asanas). It is the yoga postures that are best known here, often taught as a form of exercise or relaxation separate from the rest. Many very different styles of yoga exist, some very vigorous and demanding, some quite gentle. I couldn't be more pleased to see yoga becoming so mainstream in our part of the world; I think it will increase the numbers of healthier and happier people here. But I do not recommend the strenuous forms for everyone. Older people will do best with gentle forms of hatha yoga. If you have any injuries, musculoskeletal problems, or significant medical problems, look for opportunities to learn and practice therapeutic yoga.

You can take yoga in group classes, now widely available, or find instructors to work with you individually. Most people I know enjoy group sessions, and some also practice on their own. Try to learn yoga breathing and philosophy while you're at it. They will serve you in other ways that I will discuss when I advise you about methods to protect yourself from the harmful effects of stress.

Of course, there are perfectly good non-yogic stretches as well, many that you can figure out for yourself. The advantage of learning a basic series of asanas is that they stretch and tone all the major groups of muscles. There is a repertory of yoga balance poses as well, with names like Mountain, Tree, and Warrior. Practice these under the supervision of an instructor until you master them.

To learn balance, you have many other options. There are balance boards that you stand on and inflatable exercise balls that you use for sit-ups, back extensions, and other moves. Some trainers say the latter are the most important invention of recent years for exercise; they are also quite inexpensive compared to other equipment. I use them as part of my indoor workouts and find them very useful. Just have someone supervise you until you feel secure on them in order to keep you from rolling off them and hurting yourself.

For a completely safe and effective form of balance training, I recommend tai chi, the slow-motion, patterned movements sometimes called "Chinese shadow boxing" or "swimming in air." This is what millions of Chinese do as morning exercise, and it is especially popular with the elderly, because it is gentle and graceful as well as empowering. Research shows that older people who practice tai chi are less likely to fall and less likely to suffer injury if they do fall. For this reason, some doctors I know are trying to introduce this form of exercise into nursing homes and assisted-living facilities.

You can learn tai chi in classes or from private instructors. The basic movements look deceptively simple and, in fact, are quite easy to learn at a beginner's level. Real mastery of them requires regular practice over time. Tai chi is actually a "soft" martial art, whose main purpose is to move life energy *(chi* or *qi)* around the body in order to increase vitality and promote health and longevity. I have met long-time students of it who do indeed appear unusually vital and healthy for their age.

I will close this chapter with a few words about obstacles that keep people from getting enough of the right kinds of physical activity as they get older. When I ask sedentary folks why they are not more active, here are the answers I get most frequently along with my responses to them:

I don't have time for it. Physical activity is one of the most important investments you can make in long-term health and healthy aging. It has to be a priority. The actual time you need to spend is not that great: thirty to forty-five minutes a day of aerobic activity most days, thirty minutes of strength training two or three times a week, and maybe the same number of minutes for flexibility and balance training. If you can combine some of this with ordinary activity like house- or yard work or walking to work or shopping, the time requirement is even more manageable. When you establish these routines and see and feel the results, you will look forward to this time and come to enjoy it.

I'm too old to start. At whatever age you commit to regular physical activity, the benefits will accrue. It is never too late to start.

I don't know how. Read books, watch videos, work with trainers, take classes. You already know how to walk and stretch. All of the forms of activity described above are easy to learn.

I just don't like it. Most people who are not in the habit of exercising have to fight initial inertia. The inactive body can be lazy and sluggish. Most people who stick with routines of physical activity soon find them rewarding. They make you feel better, physically and emotionally, in part, perhaps, because of endorphin release and changes in metabolism. That has certainly been my experience. I did not take up regular physical activity until my late twenties, when I began to practice yoga, walk, hike, cycle, and swim. Now, if circumstances prevent me from doing my routines even for a day, I don't feel quite right; the day feels incomplete. And even if I feel sluggish when I start my aerobic exercise, it quickly becomes pleasurable. That will be your experience, too, if you just do it.

12

BODY V: REST AND SLEEP

In addition to adequate and proper physical activity, the human body needs adequate and proper rest and sleep. Most children and young adults have no problem getting them. Older people often do.

The few memories I can retrieve of nursery school and kindergarten more than half a century ago are of afternoon naps after milk (which I didn't like) and cookies (which I did), curled up on a blanket on the floor of a classroom, often in a patch of sunlight coming through a window. It was so easy then to nap and wake up refreshed. I've had to relearn that process in my sixties—without the cookies.

When I was in college—uninformed about the importance of physical activity and still leading a sedentary life—I would often come home from classes, sit down to read some assigned text, and find myself fighting off the urge to fall asleep. I would read the same sentence over and over as my mind clouded and jerk my head up when it fell forward into semiconsciousness. If I did fall asleep in this position for even a few minutes, I woke up groggy and angry with myself for not being able to concentrate. I just could not allow my brain the brief afternoon nap it wanted. I came to associate these "sleep attacks," as I called them, with inefficient study habits. The more I fought them off, the more they plagued me, and this pattern continued through medical school and most of my adult life. So I tried not to read in the afternoon, especially if I was near a comfortable chair or sofa. And always when I did fall asleep in this situation, I had bizarre dreams, sometimes with unpleasant out-of-body experiences, followed on waking by lethargy and grogginess that lasted a long time.

My study of the literature on sleep and my discussions with sleep experts have convinced me of the value of napping. People who nap generally enjoy better mental health and mental efficiency than people who do not. The quality of their nighttime sleep tends to be better as well. The timing and duration of naps are important: too much, too often, or at the wrong time of day can be counterproductive, but, generally, napping is a good thing.

I think my problem was interference from my thinking mind, which had developed a negative attitude about daytime sleeping, probably the result of incorporating the work ethic I got from family, schools, and society. Because I fought my body's desire for afternoon naps, my experience of them was unpleasant. I am happy to report that has changed. My schedule does not permit me to nap every day, but if I feel a pull toward afternoon sleep, I now take the time to lie down and enjoy it. Usually, I wake in ten to twenty minutes feeling refreshed, without any of the strange dreams or hallucinations of the past. Also, I am delighted that I can take productive naps sitting up in cars, trains, and airplanes. I do especially well on airplanes, almost always falling asleep during taxiing for takeoff and waking up once airborne. It makes the airplane experience less unpleasant.

Napping is just one way of taking care of the body's need for rest. You can also lie in a hammock or just stare into space. The essence of rest is *not doing*—that is, being passive on both the physical and mental levels. Many women I know get their rest by lounging in warm baths. (I will write about relaxation and stress protection in the next chapter; it seems to me that indulging in the bath properly belongs there.) How do you rest, if you do? Try to understand that our culture works actively against the whole concept. It bombards us with stimulation in more and more places and times. When I'm waiting to board a flight in an airport, I often can't get away from television monitors broadcasting the news, and in more and more hotel elevators these days, I find that I am forced to listen to commercial announcements or yet more news. Finding opportunities to rest in our society is not so easy.

Anthropologists note that in "primitive" cultures, such as the few hunter-gatherer societies left on Earth, people have much more leisure time than we do. How can that be? You would think that with all of our labor-saving devices and modern conveniences, we would be way ahead of them on that score. My own experiences with Indian tribes in the Amazon are in accordance with the anthropologists' reports. When I lived with the Cubeos, a tribe on the Río Cuduyarí in the Vaupés territory of eastern Colombia in the 1970s, I found that they devoted a great deal of time every day to leisure and rest. Of course, they tended their crops in cleared areas of the rain forest, fished the river, hunted, and took care of domestic chores, but most afternoons they spent considerable time in their hammocks, sat around chewing coca leaves and chatting with one another, and often enjoyed making music with flutes and drums. They took time to watch the beauty of Amazonian sunsets and contemplate the spectacular night skies and appeared to feel no guilt or conflict about any of this. We may have made progress in other areas of life but not in this one.

The body needs rest, both to balance physical activity and

to recharge the mind. Being passive, taking in your surroundings without reacting, and simply not doing anything for a time are valuable and necessary for optimum health and healthy aging. If you are not now satisfying that need, think about how you can.

The need for sleep is much more obvious: go without it, or get sleep of insufficient quality, and you are soon unable to function. Here, again, aging brings change and challenges.

We all know how difficult it is to rouse sleeping children. It is astonishing that you can carry them about, move them, and make noise in their presence without waking them. Other early memories I have are of being in the family car at night at the end of a long trip—to dinner at grandparents' or to the New Jersey shore—being barely aware of arriving at home and being carried from car to bed, wanting only to stay unconscious. Throughout grade school and probably into high school, I slept long and deeply every night and hated to get up in the morning, resenting being awakened by parents or alarm clocks. In college, I avoided early-morning classes and continued to indulge in deep, delicious sleep way past breakfast time.

The start of medical school when I was twenty-two changed all that. Suddenly, I had to get up at seven to attend eight o'clock lectures, a difficult adjustment and one that took most of a year. Once I got through it, however, I found that I began to wake up early even on some days when I didn't have to. This trend progressed until I found myself waking at dawn. Today, I cannot sleep past dawn: as soon as the sky starts to get light, I wake naturally, sometimes an inconvenience if I've had a late night. Interestingly, I mostly keep to this schedule even if I am away from home and am in a room without a window. I'm rather pleased with my ability to wake with the dawn. It feels natural, just what my body is supposed to be doing. (I don't believe in the concept of "night owls," by the way; I think people who sleep through the morning and are active at night have disconnected their biorhythms from the day/night cycle.)

My waking time also varies with the seasons. I am writing this just at the winter solstice and woke this morning close to seven o'clock, rather late for me. Six months from now, I'll be waking before five a.m. and will have the wonderfully cool desert morning ahead of me before the oven heat of summer comes on with the rising of the sun. Usually, I am in bed by ten, and I now find that I do best with seven hours of sleep a night rather than eight.

When I first fall asleep, I do so as easily as ever, usually within minutes of lying in bed. When I read in bed, that is a sure soporific, as good as any sedative I've tried. I rarely make it through more than a couple of pages. Only when I have something disturbing on my mind can I not fall asleep quickly. That happens rarely, but when it does, it absolutely keeps me from disengaging from thoughts and letting go of waking consciousness. And one more change I notice is that I get sleepy earlier than I used to, sometimes by eight-thirty or nine if I am having a quiet evening at home with little stimulation. I don't want to go to bed that early, because if I do, I'll get too much sleep or be up when it's still dark.

Sleep experts call this last change "advancement of the sleep phase" and note that it is a common experience of older people. I hear jokes about the "early-bird specials" offered by restaurants near big retirement communities like those in southern Florida—discounted meals for old people who want to eat dinner in the late afternoon, well before sunset. The many people who take advantage of them are going to be up at three or four, often wondering what to do with themselves in the middle of the night.

But the quality of my sleep has changed as I've aged. Around the age of thirty, I began to sleep much less deeply. Noise and other disturbances that would have had no effect on me in my teens and twenties began to wake me up. Sometimes, I could not easily get back to sleep, a definite change from my past and an annoying one. Now, as I get older, I seem to sleep even more lightly; at least, I am more conscious of my nighttime experience than I used to be. In my forties and fifties, I began to have to get up to urinate at night, another change. In a typical night, this happens once or twice, and usually I return to sleep easily.

To get advice on how to manage the changes in sleep associated with aging, I consulted Dr. Rubin Naiman, a psychologist on the clinical faculty of the Program in Integrative Medicine at the University of Arizona. He is an expert on sleep and dreaming and their contributions to health, as well as the author of an informative book, *Healing Night: The Science and Spirit of Sleeping, Dreaming, and Awakening*. When physician-fellows at the program present new patients at our clinical case conferences, it is always Dr. Naiman who reminds them to report on patients' habits of sleep and dreaming.

Dr. Naiman likes to refer to rest as "waking sleep," because the same neurochemical mechanism (an increase in the neurotransmitter GABA in the brain) may mediate both the daytime and nighttime versions. He points out that the more awake we get during the day, the better sleep we can get at night and that it is desirable to maintain this kind of variability as we go through life. In our culture, however, older people tend to lose it. "We are getting flatlined," he notes, "becoming sleepy during the day and wakeful at night."

Some of this is a general problem of modern civilization. In the not-distant past, day and night were much more sharply demarcated, and nights without mass electric lighting were darker. The coming of night brought dangers, but it also forced people to shift into a different mode of consciousness. Today, the distinction is blurred, and we can carry on daytime awareness and behavior in brightly lit homes and offices well into the night. (You can experience an extreme of this new pattern in Las Vegas, where huge, windowless casinos, blazing with light, noise, and other stimulation, completely insulate people from the natural cycle of light and dark, activity and sleep.)

Dr. Naiman argues that variation in the amount of light we are exposed to throughout the day has a major influence on the wake/sleep cycle. "Most people are underexposed to light during the day," he says. "Even on cloudy days, natural outdoor light is much brighter than what you get in a lighted room. Get outside!" He thinks we also need to get more darkness at night. The pineal gland secretes melatonin, our sleep-inducing hormone, with the onset of darkness. You can facilitate that natural process by spending an hour or so in dim light before going to bed (by wearing sunglasses if you have to) and by avoiding exposure to bright light once you have gone to bed. That means not falling asleep with the bedroom television on and not turning on the bathroom light if you have to get up to urinate.

Another of Naiman's recommendations for older people is to try to structure evening eating and social time later in the day. "Stay connected in the evening," he advises, because this was probably the natural trend in human affairs before we blurred the distinction between day and night. With the onset of darkness, people used to come together to eat and socialize, for both safety and comfort. Many retired people today do the opposite: they get together and eat dinner in the afternoon and spend time by themselves in the evening, giving their brains wrong signals about what time it is.

Naiman also pays great attention to patients' dreams. Rapid eye movement (REM) sleep—the phase of sleep associated with dreaming—decreases as we age. "REM is not equivalent to dreaming," Naiman says. "We're probably dreaming all the time; REM is a window through which we can observe dreaming." He sees dreaming as an expression of another type of consciousness, one tied to imagination and fantasy. Both Dr. Naiman and I believe it's important to access that realm. Meditation, daydreaming, and other altered states of consciousness are all windows to it. So is melatonin, which you can take as a supplement. Many people use it as a sleep aid, especially when crossing time zones; one of its effects is an increase in remembered dreams, sometimes vivid ones. Our own production of melatonin declines with age, and a number of experts, including Dr. Naiman, advocate melatonin replacement therapy for older people; I do, too, and will give you advice about it in a moment.

I have a very active dream life. Or rather, I should say I am very aware of my dreams, even if I do not recall them in detail. They are generally pleasant, often involving travel and adventures in exotic locations. Being aware of them is a source of satisfaction and gives me a sense of well-being. I take melatonin at bedtime maybe once every fourth night, more frequently if I am on the road, and I attribute the liveliness of my dreaming to that use.

Finally, Dr. Naiman offers this thought: "I'm struck by the yin-yang symbol as a perfect depiction of the ideal relationship of sleeping and waking. The dark and light portions are equal, and at the heart of each is the appearance of its opposite. The complement of a daytime nap may be a period of lucid consciousness at night." That might mean a lucid dream, in which you know you are dreaming, or some other experience of waking consciousness in the midst of the sleep cycle. Maybe it's not a bad thing to have some waking time in the middle of the night.

So here is my advice about rest and sleep for healthy aging:

- Rest is important. Think about how you get it. Make time for it: daily periods where you can be passive, without stimulation, doing nothing. Rest is as important as physical activity for general health.
- Naps are good. Try to get into the habit of napping: ten to twenty minutes in the afternoon, preferably lying down in a darkened room.
- Spend some time outdoors as often as you can to get exposure to bright, natural light. If you are concerned about the harmful effects of solar radiation, do it before ten in the morning or after three in the afternoon or use sunscreen.
- Try to give yourself some time—up to an hour—in dim light before you go to sleep at night. Lower the lighting in your house and bedroom, and if other members of the household object, wear sunglasses.
- Pay attention to sleep hygiene—all the details of lifestyle, including intake of caffeine and bedroom design, that affect the quality of sleep. When you are ready to go to sleep, try to keep your bedroom completely dark.
- To minimize early waking, try to postpone the evening meal until after dusk and schedule some kind of stimulating activity in the early evening.

- If your mind is too active when you get into bed, you will not be able to fall asleep, no matter how tired you are. It is good to know one or more relaxation techniques that can help you disengage from thoughts; see the next chapter for suggestions.
- The two best natural sleep aids are valerian and melatonin. Valerian is a sedative herb, used for centuries. You can find standardized extracts in health food stores and pharmacies. Take one to two capsules a half hour before bedtime. Valerian is nontoxic and nonaddictive but may leave some people with a fuzzy feeling in the morning. Melatonin is a hormone that regulates the wake/sleep cycle and other daily biorhythms. Only recently has synthetic melatonin become available as an over-the-counter supplement. I prefer sublingual tablets (to be placed under the tongue and allowed to dissolve); take 2.5 milligrams at bedtime as an occasional dose, making sure that your bedroom is completely dark. New evidence suggests that a much lower dose, 0.25 to 0.3 milligrams, is more effective for regular use.

   Melatonin causes an increase in dreaming in most people; a few people can't tolerate it because they get nightmares. Otherwise, it has no known side effects and even enhances immune function. (High doses—up to 20 milligrams every night at bedtime—can extend survival in people with metastatic cancer.)
- If you are unaware of your dream life, try melatonin. Writing down dreams or telling them to your bedmate or a recording device can also help you develop this awareness. Try keeping a notepad or voice recorder by your pillow.
- People vary in their need for sleep, from as little as four hours a night to as many as ten. Most require seven to eight hours, but needs tend to change over time. Gener-

ally, the amount of sleep you need decreases as you get older.

- If you do wake early, try to use the time productively. Read or write for an hour, then try to go back to sleep until morning. Think yin-yang—a period of nighttime wakefulness complements your daytime nap.

13

BODY VI: TOUCH AND SEX

I do not want to leave the subject of the needs of the body without writing a few words about touch and sex. Touch is a basic requirement for optimum health: touch-deprived babies, both animal and human, do not develop normally. This need does not diminish with age, but older people often have fewer opportunities to give and receive health-promoting physical contact. They may live alone, be infirm, or be isolated with other old and infirm people. They may be ashamed of their bodies and think that others do not want to touch them or be touched by them. They may be afraid of getting hurt by physical contact with younger, stronger people or with very active children, even their own grandchildren.

Often these ideas are unfounded, but they are completely unsurprising, given the dominance of the youth culture. Movies, television shows, and magazines generally equate attractiveness and huggability with youth, rarely with age. It will be interesting to see if the baby boomers are able to shift this cultural bias. They are a large and powerful segment of the population, known for their sense of entitlement, now approaching their senior years. They know what they want, and they make efforts to get it. I do not think

·boomers are going to settle for being marginalized, isolated, and untouched by the society at large.

In the meantime, I urge you as strongly as possible to find ways to touch and be touched as you move through life. One way, a perfectly good one, is to treat yourself to massage on a regular basis. Many forms of bodywork exist, from familiar Swedish massage to a myriad of specialized and exotic techniques. Your health insurance may even reimburse you for some of this, especially if a doctor prescribes it. Just ask. I have seen bodywork do wonders for the minds and spirits as well as the bodies of older people.

Lack of sex is not so easily remedied if one lives alone or with a partner who is no longer interested in or physically able to engage in it. Clearly, many older people have active sex lives and get as much or more pleasure from them as ever, even though the forms of their sexual activity may have changed over time. Recently, I spoke about healthy aging to a group in California. A couple in their early eighties was present, and the woman spoke up with great enthusiasm about the benefits of sex. "It's the best remedy I've found for aches and pains," she told me. "It takes my mind right off them." And, in fact, some research suggests that seniors who remain sexually active enjoy better physical and emotional health than those who do not.

The youth culture would have us believe that sexual pleasure is the birthright of the young, that old people shouldn't be thinking about sex, and that imagining old people having sex is distasteful. None of this is true. People who have been sexually active early in life often continue to be throughout life, as long as their physical health permits them to be. Changes in aging bodies often require adaptations in the mechanics of sex, however, from the requirement for vaginal lubrication in postmenopausal women to dealing with erectile dysfunction and declining sensitivity to stimulation in older men. Common medications prescribed to older people can also interfere with sexual function, including drugs for high blood pressure and depression. These problems have solutions.

The fact is that many seniors say that the capacity for sexual pleasure increases with age, even if frequency and intensity of sexual activity do not. The range of normal sexual activity, however, impressively broad at any age, remains great among the elderly. I see aging men who experience distress at loss of virility and take obsessive interest in drugs and devices to restore it as well as in much younger women. I know older women who are devoted to their vibrators and take them everywhere. But a very common pattern I hear from older couples is that desire for sexual intercourse has faded, even though desire for intimate touch has not. That is, people want to be held and cuddled by their partners and exchange pleasurable touch with them. They may still want orgasms but may not be interested in achieving them through intercourse. Absence of the sexual passion of younger days is not a problem for them, but absence of connection through loving touch would be.

The point is that sexuality changes as you grow older. If you agree that acceptance of aging is the goal, then you must work out your peace with changes in your sexual life. Here are some strategies I recommend:

- If you have sexual problems in later life (or at any point in life, for that matter), seek help—from doctors, sex therapists, or books (see Appendix B for suggestions). Good advice and good remedies exist for the common ones.
- Open communication about sexual needs, anxieties, and difficulties is important throughout life. If you are older

and living with a partner, try to express your needs, especially if they have changed. See if you can find areas of common ground where you can exchange some form of nurturing touch.

- It may be harder for single seniors to find sexual partners than it is for young singles, but it is not impossible. There are even Internet dating services for the elderly.
- Self-stimulation is always an option. I consider it a healthy practice throughout life.
- Remember that everyone is different. There are no rules for sex and aging. Pay attention to how your interests and appetites change. Try to adapt to those changes. And keep in mind that for some people diminished interest in sex can be a liberating and welcome change that aging brings. Go back and read the words of Cicero that I quoted earlier (see page 214).

14

MIND I: STRESS

I can tell you all you need to know about the effect of stress on health in one sentence. Cortisol, the adrenal hormone that mediates stress responses, is directly toxic to neurons in the part of the brain responsible for memory and emotion. If you want to minimize age-related deficits in mental function, you must know and practice strategies for neutralizing the harmful effects of stress on the brain and other organs.

Life is stressful and always has been. Eliminating stress entirely is not an option. Of course, if there are discrete sources of it in your life—a relationship, a job, a health problem—you can and should take action to try to mitigate them. But my experience is that we are subject to a kind of conservation law of stress, with the total remaining constant over time. If stress recedes in one area, it seems to increase in another. Get your finances in order, and your relationship sours. Get your relationship together, and the kids cause you grief. Straighten the kids out and learn that you have a heart problem.

Therefore, in addition to working on the problems and situations that create stress for you, do not fail to learn and practice the general techniques of stress protection that I am about to describe. Note that I do not use the term "stress reduction." The goal is to change your reaction to stress and by doing so to protect your body. You will recognize these techniques as relaxation methods; indeed, I urge you to cultivate the "relaxation response" that Dr. Herbert Benson at Harvard has researched and written about for so long. That response is a shift within the autonomic nervous system from sympathetic dominance to parasympathetic dominance.

Sympathetic nervous activity prepares us for fight-or-flight responses. It is the body/mind's way of dealing with danger, whether real or imagined, and it is absolutely necessary for survival. Like inflammation, however, it should occur only when needed and should remain within its appointed limits. Sympathetic stimulation causes the heart to beat faster, blood pressure to rise, blood sugar to rise, blood flow to shift away from the surface of the body to the core (causing cold extremities), and digestion to slow or stop. It also raises cortisol levels. Chronic overstimulation by the sympathetic nervous system, like chronic inflammation, can cause a multitude of diseases, from cardiac arrhythmias and hypertension to metabolic disturbances, endocrine dysfunction, imbalances of immunity, and gastrointestinal ailments. Obviously, it is also associated with anxiety and sleep disorders and, often, with defensiveness and isolation.

When the parasympathetic nervous system is dominant, heart rate slows, blood pressure falls, circulation is balanced throughout the body (making hands and skin warm), digestive organs work smoothly, and metabolism and immunity are optimal. The emotional experience that accompanies these physiological responses is a sense of well-being that makes empathy and real connection with others more likely.

I believe overactivity of the sympathetic nervous system

is a major cause of chronic illness and a major impediment to healthy aging. Moreover, it has been characteristic of human life in all places and all times. Modern, urban civilization does not have a monopoly on the problem. The conservation-of-stress law mentioned above holds true everywhere and all the time. If it's not saber-toothed tigers and threats of famine, it's rush-hour commutes and the evening news.

Recently, scientists demonstrated a direct correlation of objective and perceived stress on cellular aging. They measured length of telomeres, telomerase activity, and oxidative stress in white blood cells in healthy premenopausal women who were biological mothers of either a healthy child or a chronically ill child. The women who experienced more stress in their lives had shorter telomeres, lower telomerase activity, and greater oxidative stress than their less-stressed counterparts. All of these changes indicate accelerated aging and, probably, increased risk of age-related diseases. In this study the changes correlated with *perceived* stress and its chronicity (that is, duration over time); the greater the perception of stress and the longer it lasted, the more harmful it was.

You might wonder why I have put the subject of stress in the section of this book about mind, given how much I am writing about its physical effects. The reason is that mind is the locus of control of stress reactions that are mediated by the nervous and hormonal systems. The mind is where we can do something about the perception of stress. A psychologist friend of mine who is also a cancer survivor likes to say that life moves from crisis to crisis. I agree. But we have a choice as to how we react to the crises, even if we are unaware that we do. How you react to disturbing events is mostly a matter of habit. Habits can be changed.

Whatever objective stress you have to deal with, you can learn to activate the relaxation response. You can do so in many ways: by working with your breath, practicing yoga, taking biofeedback training, floating in water, or stroking a cat or dog that you love. But you have to practice whatever works for you and practice it regularly if you want to change the usual pattern of sympathetic dominance and go through life with your parasympathetic nervous system running your body more of the time.

I have already discussed the body's need for rest. Rest and relaxation are not synonymous, because the former is about non-doing, while the latter involves active techniques to influence the nervous system. Relaxation and stress protection make it easier to get rest as well as better-quality sleep. Rest and sleep are necessary but not sufficient to protect you from the harmful effects of stress.

When I take a medical history, I include these questions: "What is the major source of stress in your life?" "What do you do to relax?" "Have you ever had any relaxation training?" The answers to the first two are varied; the answer to the third is usually no. Common answers I get to the second are: "Have a drink," "Watch television," "Go on vacation," and "Work out." Let me tell you why I do not consider these good ways to protect yourself from stress.

Very many people use alcohol to unwind from a stressful day, especially at work, and as you know, many experts argue that moderate or occasional use of alcohol has beneficial effects on health and aging. The problem with alcohol is that it is addictive and toxic in amounts that many people consume. Since stress in life never goes away, if you depend on any substance to deal with it, legal or not, prescribed or over the counter, you will tend to use that substance regularly and can easily slide into excess. If you enjoy alcohol, use it—moderately, please—but try to master methods of neutralizing stress that do not involve mind-altering drugs.

Television can be relaxing, but that really depends on what you watch. A great deal of the programming is stimulating and simply fires up the sympathetic nervous system rather than calms it. That is certainly true of news and the very many shows that feature violence. Even commercials can create inner unrest rather than relaxation by making you want products you do not have and do not need or otherwise whetting your appetites. I love movies and often watch them at home in the evenings, but I am careful about what I watch and do not use movie watching as a substitute for relaxation practice.

Vacations may or may not be relaxing. Too often they create their own kinds of stress, different from those of workaday life but equally noxious. In any case, vacations happen too infrequently to help you cultivate the relaxation response on a regular basis.

As for exercise, I observe that many people use vigorous workouts as a way to defuse anger, reduce aggression that builds at work or on the roads, and improve mood. You can easily get a relaxation response after physical activity, but only if you make it happen. Otherwise, exercise can foster competitiveness and physiological responses more associated with sympathetic than parasympathetic activity. I am all for regular physical activity, as you know, but I do not use it as my way of protecting myself from stress.

Instead, here are the methods I use:

- *Breathwork*. Readers familiar with my writings know that I have long promoted the benefits of working with the breath as the simplest, most efficient way of taking advantage of the mind-body connection to affect both physical and mental health. Briefly stated, breathing straddles the mind-body interface. It is a unique function that can be completely voluntary and conscious or completely involuntary and unconscious. It offers the possibility of using the conscious mind and voluntary nerves to modify the unconscious mind and involuntary nerves, including the balance between the sympathetic and parasympathetic activity.

I have given detailed instructions on breathwork in other books and audio programs (see Appendix B), and I hope you will look those up. A specific relaxing breath technique that I urge you to learn is the following:

1. Place the tip of your tongue against the ridge behind and above your front teeth and keep it there through the whole exercise.
2. Exhale completely through your mouth, making a "whoosh" sound.
3. Inhale deeply and quietly through the nose to a count of 4 (with your mouth closed).
4. Hold your breath for a count of 7.
5. Exhale audibly through your mouth to a count of 8.
6. Repeat steps 3, 4, and 5 for a total of four breaths.

This can be done in any position; if seated, keep your back straight. Practice the exercise at least twice a day and, in addition, whenever you feel stressed, anxious, or off center. Do not do more than four breaths at one time for the first month of practice but repeat the exercise as often as you wish. After a month, if you are comfortable with it, increase to eight breaths each time.

With practice this will become a very powerful means of eliciting the relaxation response that gets more effective over time. It is a tonic for the nervous system, shifting energy from the sympathetic to the parasympathetic system, with many physiological benefits: lowered blood pressure and heart rate, increased circulation to the extremities and skin, and improved digestion. (Presumably, it will also decrease oxidative stress, increase telomerase activity, and help preserve telomere length in your cells.) It can also help you gain better control over your emotions and cravings.

Some general principles of breathwork are: make your breathing slower, deeper, quieter, and more regular whenever you think about it; deepen the exhalation phase of breathing by squeezing more air out of the lungs at the end of each breath (again, whenever you think about it); and keep your attention on the breath more of the time. Obvious advantages of this kind of practice are that it requires no equipment, is free, and can be done anywhere. It is the most cost- and time-efficient relaxation method I have discovered, and I teach it to all patients who consult me as well as to all health professionals I train.

- *Meditation.* I have practiced sitting meditation for many years. My practice is simple. When I awake from sleep, after washing my face and brushing my teeth, I sit with my back straight and my legs comfortably crossed, and try to keep my attention on my breathing and on sensations arising from my body for fifteen to twenty minutes. During the day, I drop into the same state for a few minutes here and there whenever I remember to do so, as a way of being mindful, of bringing full consciousness to the present moment. I believe this practice has helped me control mood swings and buffered me from depression in addition to neutralizing the effects of stress and increasing my effectiveness in various spheres of activity, from preparing food to public speaking. It has also made me more aware of my unconscious life, including intuition and dreaming.

Meditation is nothing other than focused attention, directed inward or outward—to the breath, for instance, which is probably the most natural object of meditation, or to an external visual focus or a silently spoken word or phrase. Meditation need not have any association with religious practices, Western or Eastern, and can be done by oneself or with others. You can learn basic meditation technique from books or attend groups or retreats for more intensive training. However you learn it, it does you no good unless you practice it on a regular basis. The time commitment need not be great. You will find suggestions for instructional materials on meditation in Appendix B.

- *Visualization.* A number of mind-body therapies take advantage of the power of visual imagination to affect the body and promote relaxation. I often refer patients to hypnotherapists and guided imagery practitioners who do this kind of work and see good clinical results. A basic technique of these therapies is to ask people to imagine actual places from past experience where they have felt supremely happy, secure, and peaceful. That might be a beach, a forest glade, or a room in the house one grew up in. The instruction is then to picture yourself in that scene, making all the sense impressions as sharp as possible. Where would you go in a guided imagery session? I go to a pool in a little canyon in the national park near my desert home, a place I visit frequently in real life and often meditate in.

This is another efficient way to activate the relaxation

response. Like breathwork, it makes use of a capacity that all of us have, that requires no equipment and costs nothing. Really, it is an extension of daydreaming and fantasizing, activities that our culture deems unimportant at best. We tend to regard fantasizing as time wasting and often tell daydreaming children to pay attention. They *are* paying attention—to internal reality rather than external reality—and it is through the doorway of the visual imagination that we have access to the relaxation response and its many beneficial effects on health and aging. I recommend cultivating this capacity, on your own, with a therapist, or by using books and audioprograms like those listed in Appendix B.

- *Bodywork.* In the previous chapter, I mentioned bodywork as a way of satisfying the need for physical contact, something I consider essential for optimum health and healthy aging. Here I want to make you aware of another potential of bodywork: it can evoke a powerful relaxation response.

  When I get a good massage, I almost always shift out of normal waking consciousness into an altered state that borders on waking and sleep, sometimes drifting over the edge into light sleep, then coming back to some awareness of my body, the room, and the hands of the bodyworker. A defining characteristic of this state is passivity. Given all the ways in which I am active through the hours of the day, both physically and mentally, I find it most welcome to surrender to passivity and let someone else manipulate my body. It is not the same as lying in a hammock or on a beach and resting, which can also be enjoyable. Rather, it seems to me that it is the conscious decision to turn over control to someone else that elicits the relaxation response and reminds me of a way of being

that feels important to cultivate. I can't get a good massage all the time, and neither can most people, but I recommend it as a way of becoming familiar with the
process of letting go that helps change the perception of
stress.

These are methods of stress protection that I use. There
are many other possibilities, from listening to music to being
in nature, and it is good to have more than one method in
your repertory of relaxation strategies. In the previous chapter, I mentioned the bath as a possibility. Like most men I
know, I take showers frequently and baths rarely, but I
know many women who use the bath as a main method of
neutralizing stress at the end of the day, making a ritual of it
with candles, music, and scented oils. I'm sure I loved baths
as a child, but most of the bathtubs I got into as an adult did
not seem designed for my body. It was not until I went to
Japan that I discovered the benefits of soaking in hot water
without being cramped in a typical Western tub. I have tried
to re-create that experience in my home, experimenting with
wood-fired, gas-fired, and even (in southern Arizona) solar-
heated hot tubs. I have not yet succeeded in re-creating the
Japanese experience, but I'm working on it.

I would like you to take an inventory of your life in order
to identify the ways that you activate and cultivate the
relaxation response. Remember, this needs to be done regularly and consciously. Only then will it be available to you
when the inevitable next crisis comes. It is up to you to
change your perception of the stress that all of us experience
in order to keep it from subverting your health and keeping
you from aging gracefully.

15

MIND II: THOUGHTS, EMOTIONS, ATTITUDES

Your thoughts, emotions, and attitudes are key determinants of how you age. Let me explain some of their influences on health and the aging process, then give you suggestions for moving them in better directions.

Thoughts (with a contribution from visual images) are primary sources of emotions, behavior, and (over time) of attitudes about ourselves and the world we live in. Most bad moods, most feelings of sadness and anxiety, are rooted in thoughts and habitual patterns of thought. We tend to be unconscious of the connection and untrained in ways to affect it.

The most common forms of emotional imbalance—depression and anxiety—are so common that they can properly be called epidemic. They affect people of all ages, including a large percentage of the elderly population, and certainly compromise quality of life and interfere with healthy aging. Doctors manage them with drugs, antidepressants, and antianxiety agents, the key word here being "manage." These drugs suppress depression and anxiety; they do not cure them or get to their roots. I support the use of psychiatric drugs for the short-term management of severe conditions, recognizing that depression can be life threatening and anxiety disabling, but I encourage both patients and doctors to be aware of alternative measures. The drugs can be toxic, can produce dependence, and may change brain chemistry in ways that increase rather than decrease the likelihood of emotional problems in the future.

Depression is often rooted in habitual thoughts of worthlessness and isolation, anxiety in thoughts of being out of control or incapable of responding to the daily challenges that life brings. As you age, susceptibility to this kind of thinking can easily increase. In a youth-oriented culture, older people often take on the belief that the worth of life declines with age and find themselves isolated with other old people. Inevitably, your aging body will fail you, forcing you to cut back on the activities of youth, leaving you less in control and more fearful.

I observe that old people often torment themselves with three general concerns: (1) they don't want to suffer; (2) they don't want to be burdens to others; (3) they want the remainder of their lives to be meaningful. These are real issues in later life, and they should be faced rather than obsessed over. The first one requires that you sit down with your doctors and with your family and discuss just what you want and do not want done for you in case you develop a life-threatening illness or are otherwise incapacitated. The decisions you come to should be put in writing and communicated to all who may be involved in your care. The second requires similar advance preparation, in this case with lawyers, family, and financial planners. The third puts more responsibility on you—to think about what activities might enrich your life and increase your sense of self-worth. It may be that service work of some kind or some form of creative expression will do it for you. Instead of ruminating about the emptiness of life, find something to do.

Conventional psychotherapy can make people aware of the thought patterns that give rise to emotional problems but rarely helps people change them, hence the continued popularity of suppressive medications. I consider it important to learn how to change counterproductive thought patterns. If you do not, you remain at risk for depression and anxiety, both of which are obstacles to healthy aging. Depression can sabotage motivation to treat your body well; it interferes with eating right and getting proper physical activity and sleep, for example, and it can directly lower immunity. Anxiety is associated with increased activity of the sympathetic nervous system, which blocks the relaxation response.

Changing habits of thought requires conscious effort and practice and often outside help. The best sources of help I have found are innovative forms of psychotherapy and Buddhist psychology.

Cognitive behavioral therapy, or CBT, has become popular only in recent years. It traces its remote origins to the teachings of the Buddha and a Greek philosopher, Epictetus (about A.D. 55 to about 135), a former slave who developed a science of happiness. He taught people to live in accordance with nature, to unlearn the habit of judging everything that happens as good or bad, and to learn to distinguish what is within your power to change and what is not. "Make the best use of what is in your power, take the rest as it comes" is one quote attributed to him. Another, quite central to the subject matter of both this chapter and the previous one, is "The thing that upsets people is not what happens but what they think it means."

(A well-known expression of Epictetus's philosophy is the Serenity Prayer, attributed to the late Protestant theologian Reinhold Niebuhr [1892–1971] and much used by Alcoholics Anonymous and other self-help groups: "God, grant me the Serenity to accept the things I cannot change, Courage to change the things I can, and Wisdom to know the difference."*)

Five hundred years earlier, the Buddha taught his followers that unhappiness derives from the incessant habits of judging every experience as pleasant, unpleasant, or neutral and of trying to hold on to the pleasant ones while shunning the unpleasant. He talked much about the tyranny of the undisciplined mind, recommending meditation as a way of developing the ability to observe the process of thought without getting attached to it. Attachment to thought, in the Buddhist conception, leads to emotional imbalance and, in turn, to behavior that increases suffering.

But prayer and meditation are long-term strategies that only some of us are willing to stick with. In the 1970s, a "cognitive revolution" in psychotherapy incorporated the above ideas into modern psychology and inspired the development of practical methods of implementing them. The result is that technologies now exist to help people change their patterns of thought and the emotions and behavior that derive from them. (By "technologies," I mean therapeutic strategies like CBT, not the use of devices.) Moreover, these new forms of psychotherapy are effective—as effective as the latest psychiatric drugs in many studies—and they work quickly, not requiring the commitments of time and money that older forms of talk therapy do.

One prominent exponent of the new psychology is Mar-

---

*A friend recently sent me a relevant parody titled the Senility Prayer: "God, grant me the senility to forget the people I never liked anyway, the good fortune to run into the ones I do, and the eyesight to tell the difference."

tin E. P. Seligman, a professor of psychology at the University of Pennsylvania and author of the classic work *Learned Optimism*. Seligman studied differences between persons prone to depression following setbacks in life and those who bounced back from them. He found the critical difference to be in "explanatory style"—how people explain rejections and defeats to themselves. Pessimists interpret them as confirmation of their own failings and lack of worth, while optimists do not see them as permanent and do not let them affect their sense of self-worth. Seligman's most important finding was that this difference is not just a matter of how people are but rather how people have learned to interpret their experience. Optimism can be learned. And optimists do better than pessimists in almost every aspect of life, including how well their immune systems function.

The process of learning to be optimistic begins with identification of self-defeating thoughts. This is most efficiently done with the help of a trained cognitive therapist. Once you are aware of habits of thought that lead to negative emotions, you can begin to substitute other ones. For example, whenever you notice yourself ruminating on a theme like *I am worthless and this latest setback just confirms it*, you can consciously substitute *This setback is just something that happened; I will get through it, because I am capable and resilient*. The theory behind this work is simple: it is impossible to hold opposite thoughts in mind at the same time, and the impact of a negative thought on feelings can be canceled by thinking a positive one. As you practice the substitution of positive thinking for negative thinking, it will gradually become the dominant habit. This is the cognitive part of CBT. Behavioral therapy can then show you how to change your behavior based on the new ways of thinking.

Psychotherapists, even those steeped in the new psychology, tend to pay more attention to thoughts than to images in the mind, but my experience is that images have at least as much power to call forth emotions and influence behavior and can be dealt with in the same way. That is, the impact of negative images can be neutralized by consciously calling up positive ones, like those you might use in the visualization work described in the previous chapter.

George Lakoff, a professor of cognitive science and linguistics at the University of California, Berkeley, has written about his experience of the terrorist attacks on the World Trade Center on September 11, 2001, in his insightful book *Don't Think of an Elephant!*:

> I now realize that the image of the plane going into South Tower was for me an image of a bullet going through someone's head, the flames pouring from the other side like blood spurting out. It was an assassination. The tower falling was a body falling. . . . The image afterward was hell: ashes, smoke and steam rising, the building skeleton, darkness, suffering, death. . . . By day the consequences flooded my mind; by night the images had me breathing heavily, nightmares keeping me awake. Those symbols lived in the emotional centers of my brain.

This is a graphic description of the power of images in the mind and their link to emotions. I can think of many patients I have worked with who have needed to change images they retained, images that stirred up fear and blocked healing. One was a young man with autoimmune disorders that targeted his platelets and red blood cells, causing episodic anemia and bleeding problems. He became critically ill after a serious auto accident, a head-on collision in which an oncoming driver crossed into his lane. The patient felt that it was a suicidal act; the last thing he saw before the impact was the face of the other driver with a frightening fixed grin on her face. She was killed, and his passengers were injured. Although he came through relatively unscathed physically, the psychological trauma of the event—symbolized by that image—activated his autoimmunity with a vengeance. He was unable to erase the image from his memory, and whenever it came up he would relive the terror of the accident. It kept him in a state of mind-body imbalance that fueled his autoimmune disease.

This patient learned the hard way that you cannot get rid of a negative image by trying not to see it, any more than you can get rid of a negative thought by trying not to think it. (Hence the title of George Lakoff's book.) Trying not to focus on images and thoughts you do not want only puts more mental energy into them, making them stronger and more persistent. The only strategy that works is to put energy into their opposites, into images and thoughts that are incompatible with the undesired ones and that evoke opposite feelings. Through guided imagery training, my patient learned to call up an image of a place where he felt secure and happy whenever the visual memory of the accident started to intrude on his consciousness. He practiced this faithfully, and as the unwanted image and its linked emotions faded, his disease remitted.

Here are a few suggestions for managing this aspect of mind as part of a program for healthy aging:

- Learn to identify habitual thoughts and images that produce feelings of sadness or anxiety, particularly those about the process of aging and changes in your body and appearance. If you find this hard to do on your own, consider working with a cognitive therapist, even for just a few sessions. It can be an effective short-term strategy for improving mental health.

- Do not try to stop negative thinking or imagery. Instead, practice substituting positive thoughts and images that evoke feelings of happiness and security.
- Remember that it takes practice to change mental habits. Just keep at it.

Over time, mental habits create attitudes that character-ize our ways of looking at life and interpreting our experi-ence of aging. I want to call your attention to two attitudes that I associate with healthy aging: flexibility and humor.

I have already written about the desirability of cultivating flexibility of the body, by stretching or doing yoga, for instance. The more physically flexible you are, the less you will be bothered by the routine aches and pains of aging and the less likely you will be to suffer serious injury if you fall. There is an analogous quality of flexibility of the mind that can protect you from being thrown off balance by the changes of growing older.

Here is an example of what I mean. The older you get, the more likely you are to experience loss—loss of parents, of family, of friends, of mates, of companion animals, of youth and youthful attractiveness, of sensory acuity, of indepen-dence, of body functions, possibly even of body parts. Any loss can remind you of all losses, plunging you into grief and despair. But recall the fundamental teaching of Epictetus: "The thing that upsets people is not what happens but what they think it means." He is pointing to a truth of highest importance: we have a choice as to how we interpret our experience, as to what meaning we assign to it.

Buddhist psychology also directs our attention to this

potential for choice. It aims to help us experience greater freedom in assigning meaning to what happens through the unlearning of old habits and the practice of new ones. I have watched the successful incorporation of one meditation technique derived from the Buddhist tradition, mindfulness-based stress reduction (MBSR), into medical settings to help the chronically ill improve quality of life and better deal with symptoms that medical treatment cannot change. MBSR is particularly effective with chronic pain, whatever its cause. As patients learn and practice the technique, they have the actual experience of increased freedom in interpreting their sensations. Even though they are experiencing pain, the mind can learn to regard it in a new and different way, one that decreases the stress and anxiety it generates. Then, as one is able to stop defending against the pain, the experience of pain often changes for the better.

This is the magic of which the mind is capable. Knowing it exists and knowing how to take advantage of it are most useful—I would say essential—for healthy aging.

Humor is a related attitude that helps reassign meaning to experience, one that my mother considered vital to graceful aging and maintained even through her final decline. It is a way of seeing the ridiculous side of life, the incongruities and absurdities that can make you laugh even in the midst of misfortunes, especially in the midst of misfortunes. Laughter may indeed be the best medicine and, like optimism, it can be learned. Dr. Madan Kataria, a physician from Mumbai, India, has recently started a practice called laughter yoga, in which large groups of people meet in order to laugh together as a form of physical and mental exercise. He has traveled around the world starting laughter clubs. In them, people laugh for no reason, using yogic breathing techniques at the start and not depending on jokes, comedy routines, or even a sense of humor. Soon the faked laughter turns into real laughter that goes on for fifteen to twenty minutes, leaving everyone feeling great. To be able to laugh at a bad experience—a loss, for instance—is the surest sign of healthy acceptance of it and adaptation to it.*

*One of the most affecting depictions I know of this potential of the mind is in an early (1957) film by Federico Fellini, *Le Notti di Cabiria (Nights of Cabiria)*, about a young prostitute in Rome who truly loses everything, including her life savings and love. Though devastated by what life has handed her, she is nonetheless able to find a different way of interpreting her experience and in a triumphant last scene recover her sense of humor and self-worth. Giulietta Masina, who plays the prostitute brilliantly, expresses this shift of consciousness without uttering a word—so brilliantly that many viewers regard that last scene as the greatest three minutes in the history of cinema. It is a very powerful expression of the philosophy I urge you to apply in your own life.

16

MIND III: MEMORY

"Age-related cognitive decline" is the medical term for one of the most terrifying changes that aging can bring: erosion of the mind. Recall that the MacArthur Foundation study identified maintenance of social and intellectual connectedness throughout life as a chief characteristic of successful aging, along with lifelong physical activity. If your intellect, memory, learning, use of language, concentration, and attention decline as you age, you will not be able to meet that requirement.

Of the many functions of mind, it is memory that seems most vulnerable with the passage of time. Age-related memory loss is the hallmark of what used to be called "senility" and now is more usually regarded as an early sign of Alzheimer's disease, a dreaded ailment that attacks the essence of an individual, leaving the body intact while it destroys the mind. Alzheimer's disease (AD) is the most common cause of dementia in older people. It is an age-related neurodegenerative disease of unknown cause, emphatically not a consequence of normal aging.

Of course, you will want to do whatever you can to prevent AD, especially because there is presently no cure and treatments for it are dismally inadequate. A larger issue is what can be done to preserve mental function in general, to protect ourselves from age-related cognitive decline, which some authorities do regard as part of the normal aging process, much like declining muscle mass and bone mineral density.

All of the advice I have given you in Part Two of this book will help you keep your wits about you. I have told you that AD begins with inflammation in the brain, as do other neurodegenerative diseases, and that the stress hormone cortisol is toxic to nerve cells in the part of the brain (the hippocampus) concerned with memory. Oxidative stress also undermines brain function. The anti-inflammatory diet described earlier, selected supplements, physical activity, proper rest and sleep, and neutralization of stress all work in different ways to protect the brain and mind. Another common cause of dementia is cardiovascular disease, which can deprive areas of the brain of blood supply. If you follow the recommendations in these chapters, you can reduce that risk as well.

Two factors that offer further protection against age-related cognitive decline deserve more comment. They are education and nicotine.

The more education you have, the less likely you are to develop AD or to experience age-related cognitive decline; if you do get them, they will appear later in life than in less educated people. Education thus compresses brain/mind morbidity. The reason for this seems to have to do with "neural redundancy," the total of extra connections between nerve cells in the brain.

The central nervous system is highly plastic. Its structure and function are always in dynamic flux, responding to changing needs and stimuli. Learning causes structural changes in the neural network, in how individual neurons connect to other neurons. The more learning you have had, the more connections you have in your brain, and many of these connections are redundant; that is, they are extraneous and duplicative but add to the richness and plasticity of the whole. A practical consequence is that more of such a network can be lost or damaged without loss of function, so that if some degenerative process does occur, it will take longer for it to produce symptoms of cognitive decline or dementia.

Nicotine affects brain chemistry in several ways that protect against both AD and Parkinson's disease. Some research suggests that smokers are at half the risk of nonsmokers for developing AD. The problem is that inhaled nicotine is highly addictive and has other, damaging effects on health in general and brain health in particular. It is a powerful constrictor of arteries, for example, reducing blood flow to the brain and other organs. And in cigarette smoke it comes along with a host of noxious chemicals that greatly increase oxidative stress. Research also clearly demonstrates that heavy smokers are at much greater risk for developing cognitive impairment earlier in life than nonsmokers, perhaps as early as age fifty.

What are we to make of this paradox? Certainly, no one should take up smoking for health reasons, and no one, I hope, would argue for health benefits of moderate smoking, as many legitimately do for the health benefits of moderate alcohol consumption. You should know, however, that pharmaceutical researchers are looking for less toxic analogs of nicotine that could be used for both the prevention and treatment of neurodegenerative diseases. Also, these observations about nicotine raise a more general question: are other natural products available that might stave off age-related cognitive decline?

You will find extravagant claims of this sort made for many products in health-food stores, on the Internet, and in antiaging books. In fact, there is a whole class of so-called smart drugs that have been popular for several decades. Some are prescription drugs, some are pharmaceuticals available abroad, and many are dietary supplements supposed to increase levels of neurotransmitters in the brain. Most are safe, but evidence for their efficacy is scant. I will mention three of the more promising ones here, an herbal remedy and two supplements.

Ginkgo, an extract of the leaves of the ginkgo tree *(Ginkgo biloba),* is a well-studied botanical remedy that increases blood flow to the head and has been shown to slow the progression of dementia in early-onset AD. It has a reputation as a memory-enhancing agent—some students even take it before exams—but I believe it is useful only in people with impaired circulation to the brain (as a result of atherosclerosis, for example), and, in any case, it takes six to eight weeks of continuous use to produce an effect. You can get standardized extracts of ginkgo in any health-food store. (They should contain 24 percent ginkgo flavone glycosides and 6 percent terpene lactones; the dose is 60 to 120 milligrams twice a day with food.) Ginkgo has low toxicity. It may cause mild stomach irritation and may have some anti-clotting effect, which suggests caution in using it together with prescribed blood-thinning medication.

I mentioned *acetyl-L-carnitine* (also called ALC or ALCAR), an amino acid derivative, in an earlier discussion. It is one of the two components of the rejuvenating formula that Bruce Ames developed and studied in rats. A typical statement from literature promoting sales of ALC products is "Acetyl-L-carnitine easily crosses the blood-brain barrier and its potential role in protecting neurological function is clear." In fact, clinical studies of this compound are few, and evidence from them is mixed. An objective group, the Alzheimer Research Forum, says: "There is some evidence of a modest effect of ALCAR on younger-onset AD patients [but] the evidence of ALCAR's efficacy is not very substantial or convincing. Moreover, some evidence suggests that it actually hastens the cognitive decline in some older-onset AD patients." Many people are taking ALC as a cognitive enhancer. The dose is 500 to 1,000 milligrams twice a day on an empty stomach. ALC is nontoxic, but this is an expensive regimen.

Phosphatidyl serine, or PS, is a naturally occurring lipid that is a component of cell membranes. It is considered a brain cell nutrient, and human studies using PS supplementation have reported positive effects on memory and concentration. PS may improve cognitive function in normal adults and may help reverse age-related cognitive decline. The supplement form, derived from soybeans, is readily available, though, again, not cheap. The starting dose is 100 milligrams two or three times a day; if this produces benefits after a month or more, it may be possible to go on a lower maintenance dose. PS is nontoxic, and of these three natural products it is the one I would try first.

I would not, however, rely on supplements to preserve your memory and other aspects of mental function as you age. What I would do, in addition to following all of the general lifestyle advice I have given you, is to go back to the protective effect of education and try to identify the particular kinds of learning that keep your brain and mind resilient. I meet many people who are very conscientious about physical activity. They give their bodies workouts, but they do not consider ways of working out their minds. "Use it or lose it" does not apply just to muscles; it is equally true of brain functions.

There is actually a trademarked system called Brain Gym

that claims to develop neural pathways, facilitate learning, and improve memory and concentration, but it uses physical exercises to do so. And there are many books, games, and interactive computer programs that claim to do the same, for both children and grown-ups. (Someone recently sent me a board game called GinkGo! that is supposed "to stimulate and activate the memory centers of the brain.") I have often recommended card games and word puzzles to people interested in exercising their cognitive functions.

But as I've thought more about it, I've realized that there is a particular cognitive experience that gives the most essential kind of mental workout. You can get it in various ways. I will discuss two of them: learning to use a new computer operating system and learning a foreign language.

If you use a computer, you surely know the particular kind of frustration associated with switching to a new operating system. (If you do not use a computer, think of your frustration in trying to learn.) It is maddening. Just when you had everything down and were used to the commands and formats on your screen, everything is different. You want it back the way it was. It is a real effort to make the change. It gives you a headache, causes fatigue. That feeling—the frustration, the headache, the fatigue—is exactly the kind of mental challenge that forces the neural network in the brain to change, to make more connections, to stay flexible and young. It is just like the inertia of the physical body that does not want to be worked out but is later grateful for it.

Getting used to a new computer operating system keeps you in that state for a relatively short time, usually a matter of days. Learning to use a computer if you have never used one is going to keep you there for a much longer time. It is a perfect mental challenge for older people.

At this moment in our society, there is a generational divide between the computer literate and computer illiterate. Most everyone under age sixty knows how to use one; many people over sixty do not. Among people in their seventies, eighties, and nineties, facility with computers is not so common. This is too bad for many reasons, chief among them that e-mail and the Internet provide wonderful opportunities for social and intellectual connections to people who may be physically unable to get out and about as much as they did earlier in life. Obviously, this situation will be quite different thirty years from now.

When my mother was in her mid-eighties, I tried hard to get her to use e-mail. I bought her several different devices that I thought would be easy for her to learn. I arranged for her to be tutored and had friends stop by to help whenever possible. All efforts failed. She had a mental block about that kind of technology that she could not surmount, and, eventually, she draped a decorative cloth over the computer, an announcement to me and her friends that she was done with it forever. I wish I had made the effort to train her earlier, because I know it would have enhanced her life and been good for her brain.

Try to think of kinds of learning that create that kind of intense frustration for you. Then just make yourself do them. You don't have to succeed; it is the effort that increases brain plasticity and flexibility.

This is why learning another language may be a perfect challenge for people at any age. It is an ongoing, open-ended commitment that keeps you in a continuous state of mental workout, both frustrating and rewarding. There is even fascinating research showing a direct link between bilingualism and improved brain function. We know that children raised in a bilingual environment acquire language skills more slowly than their monolingual counterparts but end up with greater mental proficiency. A recent study reports that bilingual subjects, both young and old, have faster reaction times and are better able to screen out distracting information than subjects who speak only one language. The researchers suggest that the same brain processes involved in using two languages are needed to stay focused and manage attention while ignoring irrelevant information, a facility called "fluid intelligence." Fluid intelligence is one of the first aspects of brain function to suffer in age-related cognitive decline. Therefore, proficiency at two languages ought to be protective—more so, I think, than any so-called smart drugs or supplements.

I was not exposed to a second language until I took German in high school—four years of old-fashioned language instruction that I found very hard but that allowed me to become almost fluent in that language when I spent time in Berlin during a year of travel between high school and college. Much later, I learned Spanish fairly quickly, not by studying it in school, but simply by living in a Mexican village where I was forced to speak it. I found that as I was doing so, a lot of my high school German came back, as if some language-processing center in my brain were being exercised. I am fluent in Spanish and am now determined to learn Japanese. I already have a large vocabulary and a good accent as a result of making many trips to Japan. I am confident that I would speak it passably after living there for just a couple of months and not spending time with English speakers.

By the way, I do not regard learning another language as an intellectual feat. The only talents required are the abilities to hear and to imitate sounds. After all, infants learn to speak without developed intellects and without the use of grammar books. Motivation to acquire language is essential. Infants are highly motivated, as are adults who place themselves in situations where they have to understand and make themselves understood.

To keep your brain young and protect yourself from age-related cognitive decline, learn to use a computer if you do not now use one, change your operating system frequently, and learn another language. By the way, I am not at all convinced that cognitive decline is an inevitable consequence of aging. Rather, I think most people simply do not give themselves the kinds of mental challenges that brains need to retain their functionality.

17

SPIRIT I: UNCHANGING ESSENCE

Here is an experience I have often had. I meet someone I once knew very well—say, a college friend—but have not seen in twenty years or more. This is not one of those people who looks just the same as I remember them. In fact, the changes that time has made are drastic, so great that I can barely find any resemblance between the mental picture I carried of that person and present reality. So great is the shock that social interaction is awkward. But after a few minutes, as we converse and begin to relax, I gradually adjust to the change and can again identify the person in front of me with the memory. I begin to see through the changed appearance to some unchanged essence.

This parallels another experience, one that I cited in the introduction and that I believe everyone has. Despite all the evidence to the contrary, some part of me feels the same as it always has since my earliest memories of childhood. Obviously, that is not my body, which now looks and feels different from what it was ten years ago, let alone fifty. Nor can it be my mind, which has learned so much and stored so much experience in more than half a century. I call it the unchanging essence: that part of the self that is unaffected by time. But what I'm really pointing to is spirit, the non-physical core of our being.

One of the tenets of the integrative medicine that I practice is that health and illness involve more than the physical body; good medicine must address whole persons, meaning bodies, minds, and spirits. When I have lectured on this topic in Japan, I have encountered a problem with translators. The usual translation of the English word "spirit" leads Japanese audiences to think I'm talking about ghosts, about ancestor worship and spirit possession. I'm not, of course. I'm just trying to call attention to our unchanging essence.

It is clear, however, that a great many people here as well as in Japan accord that concept no more reality than they do ghosts. If you are a materialist, if you believe that all that is real is that which can be perceived by the senses, then you will have trouble following what I have to say in this chapter and the next. Read them anyway. And then I hope you will test out the ideas in them against your own experience. They can be very useful, I believe, in coming to terms with the process of aging.

Nonmaterial reality is often the province of religion and faith. If you believe in something you cannot perceive with the senses, you will have to take it on faith. To many, faith is simply unfounded belief, belief in the absence of evidence, and that is anathema to the scientific mind. There is a great movement toward "evidence-based medicine" today, an attempt to weed out ideas and practices not supported by the kind of evidence that doctors like best: results of randomized controlled trials. This way of thinking discounts the evidence of experience. I maintain that it is possible to look at the world scientifically and also to be aware of nonmaterial reality, and I consider it important for both doctors and patients to know how to assess spiritual health.

There is a minor trend in medical education today to offer some instruction in this area. More often than not, it is offered as an elective rather than a required subject, and often it is linked to teaching about death and dying. At its best, it makes medical students aware of this other dimension of human life and gives them tools to help patients know their strengths and weaknesses, whether or not they have life-threatening illnesses.

Kathleen Dowling Singh, a transpersonal psychologist and former hospice worker, has written of the value of doing a spiritual assessment or inventory:

> It is not too late to take stock of our lives, even in the last weeks and days of terminal illness. And for those of us in the midst of life, in the apparent safety and security of our health, it is not too early. No matter how much time we have left to live, the answers to the following questions, voiced in the quiet honesty of our own hearts, provide direction to the rest of our living.
>
> Who have I been all this time?
>
> How have I used my gift of a human life?
>
> What do I need to "clear up" or "let go of" in order to be more peaceful?
>
> What gives my life meaning?
>
> For what am I grateful?
>
> What have I learned of truth and how truthfully have I learned to live?
>
> What have I learned of love and how well have I learned to love?

What have I learned about tenderness, vulnerability, intimacy, and communion?

What have I learned about courage, strength, power, and faith?

What have I learned of the human condition and how great is my compassion?

How am I handling my suffering?

How can I best share what I've learned?

What helps me open my heart and empty my mind and experience the presence of Spirit?

What will give me strength as I die? What is my relationship with that which will give me strength as I die?

If I remembered that my breaths were numbered, what would be my relationship to this breath right now?

Who am I?

Asking and answering such questions can help you connect with the core of your being and through it become more connected to others, to nature, and to higher consciousness.

Change is universal. Everything changes—everything we perceive, that is, including our thoughts, which are constantly arising, persisting for a while, and fading away. At the same time, some essence of everything is unchanging. Meditating on this paradoxical nature of reality can profoundly affect how we view ourselves and how we think about aging and death. It can be a stimulus to spiritual awakening and development, whether or not you adhere to any religion.

The best example I can give of what I mean is a story passed down through 2,500 years of history. It is the beginning of the legend of the Buddha's enlightenment, an archetypal account of an epic hero. As Joseph Campbell wrote in *The Hero with a Thousand Faces,* the hero's journey begins with a call to adventure, an event that sparks the awakening of the self. Here is Campbell's retelling of the story:

> The young prince Gautama Sakyamuni, the Future Buddha, had been protected by his father from all knowledge of age, sickness, death, or monkhood, lest he should be moved to thoughts of life renunciation; for it had been prophesied at his birth that he was to become either a world emperor or a Buddha. The king—prejudiced in favor of the royal vocation—provided his son with three palaces and forty thousand dancing girls to keep his mind attached to the world. But these only served to advance the inevitable; for while still relatively young, the youth exhausted for himself the fields of fleshly joy and became ripe for the other experience. The moment he was ready, the proper heralds automatically appeared.
>
> Now on a certain day the Future Buddha wished to go to the park, and told his charioteer to make ready the chariot. Accordingly, the man brought out a sumptuous and elegant chariot, and, adorning it richly, he harnessed it to four state horses of the Sindhava breed, as white as the petals of the lotus, and announced to the Future Buddha that everything was ready. And the Future Buddha mounted the chariot, which was like a palace of the gods, and proceeded toward the park.

"The time for the enlightenment of the prince Siddhartha draweth nigh," thought the gods; "we must show him a sign": and they changed one of their number into a decrepit old man, broken-toothed, gray-haired, crooked and bent of body, leaning on a staff, and trembling, and showed him to the Future Buddha, but so that only he and the charioteer saw him.

Then said the Future Buddha to the charioteer, "Friend, pray who is this man? Even his hair is not like that of other men." And when he heard the answer, he said, "Shame on birth, since to every one that is born old age must come." And agitated in heart, he thereupon returned and ascended his palace.

"Why has my son returned so quickly?" asked the king.

"Sire, he has seen an old man," was the reply; "and because he has seen an old man, he is about to retire from the world."

Three more messengers continue the call. On subsequent excursions, the prince sees a sick man, a dead man, and a monk, and the effect of these four encounters is to drive him from the protected environment of the palace to renounce worldly life and seek enlightenment. The spiritual awakening of the Future Buddha began with his awareness of aging, with the realization that life is not static but ever changing and that the end result of that change is senescence and decay.

The story hints at a potential of aging seldom acknowledged: contemplation of it can catalyze the awakening of the self and propel spiritual growth and development. One way it does so is by forcing us to consider what aspect of the self does not change, even as time alters our bodies and minds. Furthermore, awareness of aging and mortality can inspire us to engage more with life, to live it to the fullest, and to fulfill our potential for accomplishment. My personal reflection is that as I have advanced in age, I have become more productive, more focused, and more concerned with what I will be leaving behind as a legacy. By the way, it is because of this potential that I take the position I have, counseling against the denial of aging.

In *8 Weeks to Optimum Health,* I wrote out week-by-week suggestions for making changes in lifestyle that address all three components of human beings: the physical, the mental, and the spiritual. Here, at the risk of repeating myself, are some of the recommendations I made for enhancing spiritual health and well-being:

- Pay attention to your breath. Many cultures identify breath with spirit, seeing the breath cycle as the movement of spirit in the physical body. Practicing keeping your attention on the breath without trying to influence it is a way of increasing awareness of your nonphysical essence. (It is also much safer than focusing your attention on thoughts and images, which are often sources of negative emotions.) Finally, breath is the link to the basic life energy that circulates through us—what the Chinese call *qi* (chi) and yogis *prana*—and connects us to the source of universal energy. Simply minding the breath is a way of expanding consciousness beyond the ego, of experiencing transcendence.
- Connect with nature. You can do this by walking or sitting in a natural setting; a city park will do just fine. Allow yourself to slow down, drop your usual routines, and just absorb the influence of the place.
- Make a list of people in your life in whose company you feel more alive, happy, and optimistic. Make an effort to

spend more time with them. Our spiritual selves resonate with others, and that connection is healing.

- Bring flowers into your home and enjoy their beauty.
- Listen to music that you find inspirational and uplifting.
- Admire a work of art that raises your spirits: a painting, sculpture, or work of architecture.
- Reach out and try to resume connection with someone from whom you are estranged; practice forgiveness.
- Do some sort of service work. Give some of your time and energy to help others. The possibilities are endless but do not include just writing a check to charity.

When you read this list, you might not think these are spiritual activities. That might be due to the common confusion of spirituality with religion in our culture. Religious practices, like prayer and other rituals, may have spiritual purpose, but spiritual practices need not have anything to do with religion. The suggestions above are intended to help you become more aware of your spiritual self. Any activity that makes you feel more alive, more connected to others and to nature, less isolated, more comfortable with change, is beneficial. It will enhance your physical and mental health. It will help you accept the fact of your aging. It will help you to age gracefully.

18

SPIRIT II: LEGACY

Recently I learned of an ancient practice, now modernized and promoted for spiritual well-being. It is the writing of an *ethical will.*

An ordinary will or last testament mainly concerns the disposition of one's material possessions at death. An ethical will has to do with nonmaterial gifts: the values and life lessons that you wish to leave to others.

In many cultures, elders, sages, and saints have saved some of their pithiest teachings for students and disciples gathered at their deathbeds. Hindu saints, Zen masters, and rabbis have been particularly good at this sort of thing; many of their last words have been written down for posterity. Formal documents that sum up acquired wisdom as the end of life approaches are also found in many cultures but are most associated with Jewish tradition. Jewish ethical wills almost a thousand years old are preserved, and the practice of writing them appears to go back at least a thousand years before that.

I have looked over examples of this literature from Jewish communities in Europe from the past few hundred years. Some of them are moving, some tedious, some funny. Most of the old ethical wills I have read are the words of dying men urging their children, particularly their sons, to lead pious lives and hold true to the values of their fathers. Some are hortatory, some querulous. "Thou knowest, my son! the trouble and expense that I endured for the marriage of thy elder and younger sisters," one father begins his advice. Here are a few other quotations I enjoy:

> Therefore, my son! Exert thyself whilst still young, the more so as thou even now complainest of weak memory. What, then, wilt thou do in old age, the mother of forgetfulness? Awake, my son! from thy sleep; devote thyself to science and religion.

> My son! Drink no water that has been left uncovered overnight. Many pitfalls exist in the world, and in them men are caught, as birds are trapped in a snare.

> Show honor to thyself, thy household, and thy children by providing decent clothing, as far as thy means allow; for it is unbecoming for any one, when not at work, to go shabbily dressed. Spare from thy belly and put it on thy back!

> These are the things which my sons and daughters shall do at my request. They shall go to the house of prayer morning and evening. . . . So soon as the service is over, they shall occupy themselves a little with the Torah, the Psalms, or with works of charity. Their business must be conducted honestly, in their dealings with both Jew and Gentile.

> And this too let me impress upon you all. The penalty for leaving a promise undone is greater than a man can bear!

Much of this sounds quaint, dated, and irrelevant to contemporary life. How interesting, then, that the ethical will is currently making a strong comeback—not necessarily among Jews, not necessarily associated with death and dying—and is of great contemporary relevance, particularly for those of us concerned with making sense of our lives and the fact of our aging.

A Web site dedicated to ethical wills advises people to think of this kind of work as writing "a love letter to your family." (I would broaden the concept of family to include friends and the community at large.) It also tells us that "ethical wills are a way to share your values, blessings, life's lessons, hopes and dreams for the future, love, and forgiveness. . . . Today, ethical wills are being written by people at turning points in their lives: facing challenging life situations and at transitional life stages. They are usually shared with family and community while the writer is still alive."

I can think of no better way to end this book than to recommend that you undertake the composition of an ethical will. No matter how old you are, it can be an exercise that will make you take stock of your life experience and distill from it the values and wisdom that you have gained. You can then put the document aside, read it over as the years pass, and revise it from time to time as you see fit. Certainly, an ethical will can be a wonderful gift to leave to your family at the end of your life, but I think its main importance is what it can give you in the midst of life.

I would like to share with you some of the content of my own ethical will, as it stands when I am sixty-two years old, on the verge of becoming an elder, at the point in life when medical science would lead me to expect the beginning of age-related decline in physical and mental health.

I have learned to rely greatly on intuition, on my inner sense of right and wrong, truth and falsehood. I have cultivated the ability to hear that inner voice, and I test it constantly against my experience and external sources of information. I believe everyone is intuitive; regrettably, our educational systems do not teach us to use that faculty. You must learn it on your own.

I have always been skeptical of certainty, whether in science, medicine, or any other field of knowledge. Whenever some authority tells me, "This is how it is," my mind always looks for other interpretations of the data. I am comfortable with uncertainty, and I advise you to learn to be as well. We live in an uncertain universe.

Either-or formulations of reality make me uneasy. I much prefer *both-and* formulations. They may seem awkward at first, but they open up many more possibilities and make life more interesting. Try them out. (For example, I try to own both the light and dark aspects of my nature, just as I try to enjoy both day and night.)

Travel and experience of other cultures have profoundly influenced my worldview. I believe in multiple realities. It is possible to construct different pictures of reality from our sensory data, all of which can be internally consistent and valid. It takes effort to cast off the blinders of your own culture and become aware of this truth.

It is important to live in harmony with nature. Many people I meet are fearful of nature, regarding it as fundamentally hostile. I am sorry to say I encounter this attitude a lot in my own profession. Many of my medical colleagues really believe that pharmaceutical drugs are safer than herbal remedies, for example, because the drugs are known and pure. In my experience, it is just the other way around. (The percentage of plants or mushrooms or insects that can kill or seriously hurt you is very tiny; the percentage of pharmaceutical drugs that can kill or seriously hurt you is not tiny.) Nature may be complex and wild, but you want it as your ally, not your enemy.

I observe a curious and fascinating interplay between internal reality and external reality. What we carry in our heads affects and determines our experience of the outer world. A familiar example is that fear of an animal like a dog causes it to act aggressively. When you encounter things you don't like out there, it is worth trying to figure out how you can modify them by changing your perception of them or your relationship to them.

This principle clearly applies to interactions with other people. It is always worth looking for points of correspondence and similarity between yourself and others; this is the basis of compassion. I have learned that when I cannot stand something in another person, it is often a reflection of something that I dislike or have tried to disown in myself. Everything is projection until proved otherwise.

I believe in magic and mystery. I am also committed to scientific method and knowledge based on evidence. How can this be? I have told you that I operate from a *both-and* mentality, not an *either-or* one.

I believe that consciousness is primary, that it is more basic than matter or energy and that it directs evolution of the material universe. I am not interested in trying to prove this conviction or argue it with scientific materialists. The materialists believe that a blind process of natural selection has created the universe, that consciousness is just an "epiphenomenon" arising from bio-chemical and electrical activity of the brain. My way of thinking works for me and makes more sense of my experience than other beliefs I have explored.

Although I am as much subject to emotional ups and downs and dark nights of the soul as anyone else, when I am most centered and clear I have a powerful, deep, and, I'm tempted to say, *nonrational* sense that every-thing is just the way it's supposed to be, including the fact of my aging and movement toward death. I cannot explain this, but when I have it, I am less anxious, more accepting of change, more content.

Finally, I want to extend to you my blessings and wishes for graceful, healthy aging as you advance in years. I hope that you will discover and enjoy the bene-fits that aging can bring: wisdom, depth of character, the smoothing out of what is rough and harsh, the evapora-tion of what is inconsequential, and the concentration of true worth.

And, don't forget to wear decent clothing; it's not good to go around shabbily dressed.

A TWELVE-POINT PROGRAM FOR HEALTHY AGING

I thought it might be useful to condense the prescriptive advice in this book to a bare-bones list of instructions. Here they are:

1. Eat an anti-inflammatory diet.

2. Use dietary supplements wisely to support the body's defenses and natural healing power.

3. Use preventive medicine intelligently: know your risks of age-related disease, get appropriate diagnostic and screening tests and immunizations, and treat problems (like elevated blood pressure and cholesterol) in their early stages.

4. Get regular physical activity throughout life.

5. Get adequate rest and sleep.

6. Learn and practice methods of stress protection.

7. Exercise your mind as well as your body.

8. Maintain social and intellectual connections as you go through life.

9. Be flexible in mind and body: learn to adapt to losses and let go of behaviors no longer appropriate for your age.

10. Think about and try to discover for yourself the benefits of aging.

11. Do not deny the reality of aging or put energy into trying to stop it. Use the experience of aging as a stimulus for spiritual awakening and growth.

12. Keep an ongoing record of the lessons you learn, the wisdom you gain, and the values you hold. At critical points in your life, read this over, add to it, revise it, and share it with people you care about.

Glossary

Cross-referenced entries are in *italics*.

Acromegaly: A disorder marked by progressive enlargement of the head, face, hands, and feet due to excessive secretion of growth hormone in adults; enlargement of internal organs and diabetes may also develop.

Amino acids: The building blocks of proteins; simple *organic* compounds containing nitrogen.

Anabolic: Referring to the building-up phase of *metabolism* that converts small molecules to larger ones, as in *anabolic steroids*.

Anabolic steroids: Drugs that increase muscle bulk and bone density as a result of their effects on *metabolism*.

Asexual: Without sex, as in asexual (vegetative) reproduction.

Autoimmunity: A disease state in which the immune system attacks the body's own tissues.

Bariatric: Referring to body weight. Bariatric medicine is weight-loss medicine.

Beta-blockers: A class of drugs that block or inhibit some responses to sympathetic nervous system activity, widely used to treat cardiovascular disorders like *hypertension*.

Carcinogenic: Cancer causing.

Cardiovascular system: The heart and blood vessels and circulation.

Catalyst: In chemistry, a substance that accelerates a chemical reaction without itself being used up or changed.

Cellulose: The basis of vegetable fiber: a complex carbohydrate (too complex for the human digestive system to dismantle) composed of long chains of sugar molecules.

Centenarians: People aged one hundred years or more.

Chromosomes: Rodlike structures containing genetic material (DNA) in the nucleus of a cell. Human *somatic* cells have forty-six paired chromosomes; *germ cells* have twenty-three unpaired chromosomes.

Cognitive: Pertaining to the mental process of knowing, including awareness, perception, reasoning, and judgment.

Compression of morbidity: Reduction of the amount of time at the end of life spent in sickness and decline—the most important strategy for achieving healthy aging.

Cross-linking: Formation of abnormal chemical bonds between adjacent protein strands that deform the proteins, often impairing their function in the body.

Daughter cells: The products of the division (replication) of *somatic* cells. When a cell undergoes division, the result is two genetically identical daughter cells.

Dementia: The loss, usually progressive, of *cognitive* and intellectual functions, without impairment of perception or consciousness.

Distillation: The process of purifying a liquid by heating it to boiling, then cooling the vapor to condense and collect it.

Diuretics: Substances that increase the production and flow of urine.

DNA: Deoxyribonucleic acid, the genetic material common to all forms of life. Genes are segments of DNA that code for the production of specific proteins.

EBCT: Electron beam computed tomography, a diagnostic test using a fast X-ray scan to determine the presence or absence of calcium deposits in and around the coronary arteries.

Enzyme: A protein catalyst of biochemical reactions.

Estrogen: Any substance, natural or synthetic, that exerts biological effects typical of female sex hormones. Estrogens stimulate secondary sex characteristics and control the menstrual cycle in women.

Fermentation: A chemical change, facilitated by an *enzyme,* by which complex *organic* compounds are split into simpler compounds; the process by which microorganisms digest and obtain energy from food molecules without using oxygen.

Food chain: The sequence of organisms in which those above feed on those below.

Free radical: An unstable, highly reactive atom or atom group carrying an unpaired electron.

Genome: The complete sequence of genes distinctive of an organism. The human genome contains 20,000 to 25,000 genes, all the information needed to make a new human being.

Germ cells: Eggs and sperm (ova and spermatozoa), as distinct from *somatic* cells.

Glucose tolerance: The ability of the body to clear glucose from the blood, usually measured by giving an individual a quantity of glucose solution to drink, measuring blood glucose at intervals thereafter. Impaired glucose tolerance is a characteristic of *metabolic syndrome* and diabetes.

Glycation: A chemical reaction between sugars and proteins. In living organisms, glycation is abnormal and results in toxic products that can accelerate aging.

Glycemic load: A measure of the impact of a carbohydrate food on the body. It takes account of the amount of carbohydrate in a serving of the food and the rate at which that particular carbohydrate turns into blood sugar (glucose).

Hatha yoga: The form of yoga most familiar to Westerners; it emphasizes physical postures, called asanas.

Hayflick limit: The number of times a cell can divide (replicate). The Hayflick limit differs from species to species and corresponds with the length of *telomeres,* the end portions of *chromosomes.*

HGH: Human growth hormone, produced naturally by the pituitary gland and also manufactured by pharmaceutical companies.

Hippocampus: A structure in the brain that processes memory and emotion.

Homeostasis: The processes by which the body maintains equilibrium (balance between opposing pressures) of various functions and chemical compositions of fluids and tissues.

Hormone: A chemical substance formed in one organ or part of the body that is carried in the blood to another organ or part, where it alters body structure or function.

Hypertension: High blood pressure.

Immortalization: The process by which *malignant* cells bypass the *Hayflick limit* and gain the ability to replicate themselves indefinitely. It mostly involves activation of *telomerase.*

Inflammatory response: Localized redness, heat, swelling, and pain at the site of injury or infectious attack.

Leukotrienes: A class of *hormones* that mediate inflammation and allergic responses. The body makes them from arachidonic acid, a component of dietary fat.

Lignins: A class of long-chain chemical compounds composed of alcohol subunits that give strength to wood; lignins occur together with *cellulose* in wood and other plant fibers.

Macronutrients: Carbohydrates, fats, and proteins—foods needed in large amounts to maintain normal *metabolism* and growth.

Malignant: Cancerous; having the property of locally invasive and destructive growth and *metastasis*.

Malignant transformation: The process by which a normal cell turns cancerous. *Immortalization* is one characteristic of malignant transformation.

Metabolic syndrome: A disorder characterized by impaired *glucose tolerance,* insulin resistance, high serum triglycerides, low serum HDL (good) cholesterol, and tendencies toward *hypertension* and weight gain in the abdomen.

Metabolism: The sum of chemical and physical changes occurring in living tissue whose role is to release or provide energy.

Metabolite: Any substance that is a product of *metabolism.*

Metastasis: The spread of a disease process from one part of the body to another, as in cancer, where *malignant* cells leave their site of origin and establish new tumors in distant sites.

Micronutrients: Foods necessary in relatively small amounts to maintain normal *metabolism* and growth: vitamins, minerals, fiber, and phytonutrients.

Mitochondria: Structures (organelles) within cells where *respiratory metabolism* takes place. Mitochondria are believed to be bacteria that were captured by cells of animals in the course of evolution.

Monozygotic: Developing from one fertilized egg, as in the case of identical twins.

Organic: In chemistry, referring to compounds of carbon; in agriculture, referring to production of food without the use of chemical pesticides, fertilizers, or genetic manipulation.

Oxidation: (1) A chemical combination with oxygen. (2) A loss of electrons from an atom or compound, leaving it more positively charged.

Oxidative stress: The total pressure of *oxidation* reactions on an organism, including the production of toxic *free radicals* in the course of normal metabolism. The body requires defenses against oxidative stress in order to remain healthy.

PCBs: Polychlorinated biphenyls, a class of man-made chemical compounds, formerly used as coolants and lubricants in industrial equipment, now banned because they build up in the environment and cause harmful effects on health.

Photosynthesis: The biochemical process by which green plants use the energy of sunlight to split molecules of water and combine their atoms with carbon dioxide to produce glucose and liberate oxygen as a by-product.

Polypore: A large family of mushrooms that produce reproductive cells (spores) from a layer of tissue with many tiny holes or pores. Many are shelf fungi that grow on living or dead trees.

Polyunsaturated fatty acids (PUFAs): Component molecules of fats that have more than one double or triple bond between carbon atoms in their chains. Fats, like vegetable oils, with a high content of PUFAs are liquid at room temperature, and the more PUFAs, the colder the temperature at which the fat will begin to solidify.

Prostaglandins: A class of physiologically active substances, present in many tissues and derived from fatty acids in the diet, that mediate the *inflammatory response,* cause blood vessels to dilate and constrict, and affect involuntary muscles in various organs.

Proteolysis: The decomposition of protein.

Recombinant DNA: Altered DNA resulting from the insertion into the chain of a sequence not originally present in that chain. A technique widely used by pharmaceutical companies to turn bacteria into factories for making hormones and other desired gene products.

Respiration: (1) The exchange of oxygen and carbon dioxide in the lungs. (2) The *oxidation* of foodstuffs in cells, releasing energy and producing carbon dioxide and water.

Respiratory metabolism: The *oxidation* of foodstuffs in cells, releasing energy and producing carbon dioxide and water.

Selection bias: Distortion of research data as a result of not working with a group of subjects representative of the population under study.

Senescence: The phase of decline in the course of aging. On the cellular level, senescence is marked by the inability to replicate.

Somatic: Referring to the body. On the cellular level, referring to cells that compose the body as opposed to reproductive or *germ cells* that have half the normal number of *chromosomes.*

Soporific: An inducer of sleep.

Synergistic: Having an additive effect that is greater than the sum of the effects of the component parts.

Tannins: A large class of complex constituents of plants that have been used in the tanning of animal hides and in dyeing. They form black stains in the presence of iron, a basis for their use in inks.

Telomerase: An enzyme, absent from most normal cells, that adds length to *telomeres,* restoring the ability of *senescent* cells to replicate. It also makes malignant cells immortal.

Telomere: The end body of a chromosome, consisting of repeating short sequences of DNA code. A portion of the telomere is lost with each cell division, until the *Hayflick limit* is reached and replication ceases.

Trans fats: Deformed *polyunsaturated fatty acids* that have a jointed rather than the normal curved shape. They result mostly from treatment of edible oils with heat and chemicals.

Zygote: A fertilized egg, resulting from the combination of an egg and a sperm.

Appendix A

The Anti-inflammatory Diet

This is a summary of the specifics of a diet intended to prevent inappropriate inflammation and so reduce the risk of age-related diseases. Such a diet is also the one that I recommend to promote optimum health at any age.

GENERAL

- Aim for variety.
- Include as much fresh food as possible.
- Minimize your consumption of processed foods and fast food.
- Eat an abundance of fruits and vegetables.

CALORIC INTAKE

- Most adults need to consume between 2,000 and 3,000 calories a day.
- Women and smaller and less active people need fewer calories.
- Men and bigger and more active people need more calories.
- If you are eating the appropriate number of calories for your level of activity, your weight should not fluctuate greatly.
- The distribution of calories you take in should be as follows: 40 to 50 percent from carbohydrates, 30 percent from fat, and 20 to 30 percent from protein.
- Try to include carbohydrates, fat, and protein at each meal.

CARBOHYDRATES

- On a 2,000-calorie-a-day diet, adult women should eat about 160 to 200 grams of carbohydrates a day.
- Adult men should eat about 240 to 300 grams of carbohydrates a day.
- The majority of this should be in the form of less-refined, less-processed foods with low glycemic loads.
- Reduce your consumption of foods made with wheat flour and sugar, especially bread and most packaged snack foods (including chips and pretzels).
- Eat more whole grains (not whole-wheat-flour products), beans, winter squashes, and sweet potatoes.
- Cook pasta al dente and eat it in moderation.
- Avoid products made with high-fructose corn syrup.

FAT

- On a 2,000-calorie-a-day diet, 600 calories can come from fat—that is, about 67 grams. This should be in a ratio of 1:2:1 of saturated to monounsaturated to polyunsaturated fat.
- Reduce your intake of saturated fat by eating less butter, cream, cheese, and other full-fat dairy products, unskinned chicken, fatty meats, and products made with coconut and palm kernel oils.
- Use extra-virgin olive oil as a main cooking oil. If you want a neutral-tasting oil, use expeller-pressed, organic canola oil. High-oleic versions of sunflower and safflower oil are acceptable also, preferably non-GMO (genetically modified organism).
- Avoid regular safflower and sunflower oils, corn oil, cottonseed oil, and mixed vegetable oils.
- Strictly avoid margarine, vegetable shortening, and all products listing them as ingredients. Strictly avoid all products made with partially hydrogenated oils of any kind.
- Include in your diet avocados and nuts, especially walnuts, cashews, and almonds and nut butters made from them.
- For omega-3 fatty acids, eat salmon (preferably fresh or frozen wild or canned sockeye), sardines packed in water or olive oil,

herring, black cod (sablefish, butterfish), omega-3 fortified eggs, hemp seeds, flaxseeds (preferably freshly ground), and walnuts; or take a fish oil supplement (see below).

PROTEIN

- On a 2,000-calorie-a-day diet, your daily intake of protein should be between 80 and 120 grams. Eat less protein if you have liver or kidney problems, allergies, or autoimmune disease.
- Decrease your consumption of animal protein except for fish and reduced-fat dairy products.
- Eat more vegetable protein, especially from beans in general and soybeans in particular. Become familiar with the range of soy foods available to find ones you like.

FIBER

- Try to eat 40 grams of fiber a day. You can achieve this by increasing your consumption of fruit, especially berries, vegetables (especially beans), and whole grains.
- Ready-made cereals can be good fiber sources, but read labels to make sure they give you at least 4 and preferably 5 grams of bran per one-ounce serving.

PHYTONUTRIENTS

- To get maximum natural protection against age-related diseases, including cardiovascular disease, cancer, and neurodegenerative disease, as well as against environmental toxicity, eat a variety of fruits, vegetables, and mushrooms.
- Choose fruits and vegetables from all parts of the color spectrum, especially berries, tomatoes, orange and yellow fruits, and dark leafy greens.
- Choose organic produce whenever possible. Learn which conventionally grown crops are most likely to carry pesticide residues (see www.foodnews.org) and avoid them.
- Eat cruciferous (cabbage-family) vegetables regularly.
- Include soy foods in your diet.

- Drink tea instead of coffee, especially good-quality white, green, or oolong tea.
- If you drink alcohol, use red wine preferentially.
- Enjoy plain dark chocolate (with a minimum cocoa content of 70 percent) in moderation.

VITAMINS AND MINERALS

- The best way to obtain all of your daily vitamins, minerals, and micronutrients is by eating a diet high in fresh foods with an abundance of fruits and vegetables.
- In addition, supplement your diet with the following antioxidant cocktail:
  > Vitamin C, 200 milligrams a day
  > Vitamin E, 400 IU of natural mixed tocopherols
  > (d-alpha-tocopherol with other tocopherols, or, better, a minimum of 80 milligrams of natural mixed tocopherols and tocotrienols)
  > Selenium, 200 micrograms of an organic (yeast-bound) form
  > Mixed carotenoids, 10, 000 to 15,000 IU daily.
- In addition, take daily multivitamin-multimineral supplements that provide at least 400 micrograms of folic acid and at least 1,000 IU of vitamin D. They should contain no iron and no preformed vitamin A (retinol).
- Women should take supplemental calcium, 500–700 milligrams a day, preferably as calcium citrate, depending on their dietary intake of that mineral; men should get no more than 700 milligrams of calcium a day from all sources and do not need to supplement.

OTHER DIETARY SUPPLEMENTS

- If you are not eating oily fish at least twice a week, take supplemental fish oil, in capsule or liquid form, 1 to 2 grams a day. Look for molecularly distilled products certified to be free of heavy metals and other contaminants.
- Talk to your doctor about going on low-dose aspirin therapy, one or two baby aspirins (81 or 162 milligrams) a day.

- If you are not regularly eating ginger and turmeric, consider taking these in supplemental form (see Appendix B).
- Add Co-Q-10 to your daily regimen: 60 to 100 milligrams of a softgel form taken with your largest meal.
- If you are prone to metabolic syndrome, take alpha-lipoic acid, 100 to 400 milligrams a day.

WATER

- Try to drink 6 to 8 glasses of pure water a day or drinks that are mostly water (tea, very diluted fruit juice, sparkling water with lemon).
- Use bottled water or get a home water purifier if your tap water tastes of chlorine or other contaminants or if you live in an area where the water is known or suspected to be contaminated (see Appendix B).

WEB SITE

For more information on the Anti-inflammatory Diet, including meal planning, shopping guides, and recipes, see www.healthyaging.com.

Appendix B

Suggested Reading, Resources, and Supplies

BOOKS

Herbert Benson, *The Relaxation Response* (New York: HarperTorch, 1976)

Wayne Booth, *The Art of Growing Older: Writers on Living and Aging* (Chicago: University of Chicago Press, 1996)

Thomas R. Cole and Mary G. Winkler, *The Oxford Book of Aging: Reflections on the Journey of Life* (New York: Oxford University Press, 1994)

Ken Dychtwald, *Age Power: How the 21st Century Will Be Ruled by the New Old* (Los Angeles: Tarcher, 2000)

Leonard Hayflick, *How and Why We Age* (New York: Ballantine, 1996)

David Heber, *What Color Is Your Diet?* (New York: Regan Books, 2002)

Lana Holstein, *How to Have Magnificent Sex: Improve Your Relationship and Start to Have the Best Sex of Your Life* (New York: Three Rivers Press, 2003)

Jon Kabat-Zinn, *Full Catastrophe Living: Using the Wisdom of Your Body and Mind to Face Stress, Pain, and Illness* (New York: Delta, 1990)

Jon Kabat-Zinn, *Wherever You Go, There You Are: Mindfulness Meditation in Everyday Life* (New York: Hyperion, 1995)

Tom Kirkwood, *The Time of Our Lives: The Science of Human Aging* (New York: Oxford University Press, 1999)

Nick Lane, *Oxygen: The Molecule That Made the World* (New York: Oxford University Press, 2002)

David Mahoney and Richard Restak, *Longevity Strategy: How to Live to 100 Using the Brain-Body Connection* (Hoboken, New Jersey: Wiley, 1999)

S. Jay Olshansky and Bruce Carnes, *The Quest for Immortality: Science at the Frontiers of Aging* (New York: W. W. Norton, 2001)

David Perlmutter and Carol Colman, *The Better Brain Book: The Best Tools for Improving Memory and Sharpness and for Preventing Aging of the Brain* (New York: Riverhead Books, 2004)

Thomas T. Perls, Margery Hutter Silver, and John Lauerman, *Living to 100: Lessons in Living to Your Maximum Potential at Any Age* (New York: Basic Books, 2000)

Michael Rose, *The Long Tomorrow: How Evolution Can Help Us Postpone Aging* (New York: Oxford University Press, 2005)

John W. Rowe and Robert L. Kahn, *Successful Aging* (New York: Pantheon, 1998)

Robert M. Sapolsky, *Why Zebras Don't Get Ulcers: An Updated Guide to Stress, Stress-Related Diseases, and Coping*, 2nd ed. (New York: W. H. Freeman, 1998)

Zalman Schachter-Shalomi and Ronald S. Miller, *From Age-ing to Sage-ing: A Profound New Vision of Growing Older* (New York: Warner Books, 1997)

Martin E. P. Seligman, *Learned Optimism* (New York: Alfred A. Knopf, 1991)

David Snowdon, *Aging with Grace: What the Nun Study Teaches Us about Leading Longer, Healthier, and More Meaningful Lives* (New York: Bantam, 2002)

George E. Vaillant, *Aging Well: Surprising Guideposts to a Happier Life from the Landmark Harvard Study of Adult Development* (Boston: Little, Brown, 2003)

Andrew Weil, *Eating Well for Optimum Health: The Essential Guide to Bringing Health and Pleasure Back to Eating* (New York: HarperCollins, 2001)

Andrew Weil, *8 Weeks to Optimum Health: A Proven Program for Taking Full Advantage of Your Body's Natural Healing Power*, rev. ed. (New York: Ballantine, 2006)

Andrew Weil, *Natural Health, Natural Medicine: The Complete Guide to Wellness and Self-Care for Optimum Health*, rev. ed. (Boston: Houghton Mifflin, 2004)

Andrew Weil, *Spontaneous Healing: How to Discover and Enhance Your Body's Natural Ability to Maintain and Heal Itself* (New York: Ballantine, 2000)

Bradley J. Willcox, D. Craig Willcox, and Makoto Suzuki, *The Okinawa Program: How the World's Longest-Lived People Achieve Everlasting Health—And How You Can Too* (New York: Three Rivers Press, 2002)

Walter C. Willett and P. J. Skerrett, *Eat, Drink, and Be Healthy: The Harvard Medical School Guide to Healthy Eating* (New York: Free Press, 2002)

Rodney Yee, *Moving Toward Balance: 8 Weeks of Yoga with Rodney Yee* (Emmaus, Pa: Rodale Press, 2004)

NEWSLETTERS

Self Healing
42 Pleasant Street
Watertown, Massachusetts 02472
www.drweilselfhealing.com
800-523-3296

WEB SITES

Healthy Aging
www.healthyaging.com
This new premium Web site has been specially designed as an online companion to *Healthy Aging*. It offers the latest research and information on nutrition, fitness, stress management, and a wide range of health conditions, together with an online community, product recommendations, and interactive tools to benefit you in your unique process of aging gracefully.

DrWeil.com
www.drweil.com

Baltimore Longitudinal Study of Aging
www.grc.nia.nih.gov/branches/blsa/blsa.htm

The University of Georgia Gerontology Center
www.geron.uga.edu/centenarian_study.html

National Center for Creative Aging
www.creativeaging.org

National Institute on Aging
www.nia.nih.gov

NIH Senior Health
www.nihseniorhealth.gov/listoftopics.html

AUDIO PROGRAMS

Andrew Weil, "Breathing: The Master Key to Self Healing," *Sounds True* audio edition, 1999

Andrew Weil and Jon Kabat-Zinn, "Meditation for Optimum Health: How to Use Mindfulness and Breathing to Heal Your Body and Refresh Your Mind," *Sounds True* audio edition, 2001

DIETARY SUPPLEMENTS

I recommend and use Weil Lifestyle brand vitamins from DrWeil.com. I have developed these science-based formulations and oversee their production. Go to www.drweil.com and click on the Supplement Center or go to the Vitamin Advisor, or call 800-585-5055 for information. These products are also available at many specialty health stores under the Weil Lifestyle brand.

All of my after-tax profits from sales of these products go to a non-profit foundation that supports the development of integrative medicine. See www.weilfoundation.org.

The other products listed in this section meet my specifications for quality.

Astragalus, Dong Quai, Ginkgo Biloba, and Other Chinese Medicinal Herbs

Herbal Fortress
2106 South Big Bear Road
Coeur d'Alene, Idaho 83814
888-454-3267
www.herbalfortress.com

Medicinal Mushroom Products

Fungi Perfecti
P.O. Box 7634
Olympia, Washington 98507
800-780-9126
www.fungi.com

This company makes a product called Mycosoft Gold that I give to my canine companions.

The medicinal mushroom tonic I take daily is Host Defense Liquid, available from:

New Chapter Company
22 High Street
Brattleboro, Vermont 05301
800-543-7279
www.newchapter.info/index.html

Fish Oil Supplements

Nordic Naturals
94 Hanger Way
Watsonville, California 96076
800-662-2544
www.nordicnaturals.com

Herbs with Anti-inflammatory Properties

For supercritical extracts of ginger and turmeric, as well as the combination herbal anti-inflammatory product Zyflamend:

New Chapter Company
22 High Street
Brattleboro, Vermont 05301
800-543-7279
www.newchapter.info/index.html

Nonchlorine Pool Purification Systems

Sigma Water
1330 West Boxwood Avenue
Gilbert, Arizona 85233
800-222-7032
www.sigmawater.com

Walking Poles

Exerstrider Products, Inc.
P.O. Box 3087
Madison, Wisconsin 53714
800-554-0989
www.exerstrider.com

Water Purifiers

Purefecta
Pall Corporation
674 South Wagner Road
Ann Arbor, Michigan 48103
888-426-7255
www.pall.com/purefecta

A Note on Integrative Medicine

Integrative medicine is healing-oriented medicine that takes account of the whole person (body, mind, and spirit), including all aspects of lifestyle. It emphasizes the practitioner-patient relationship and makes use of all appropriate therapies, both conventional and alternative.

I founded and continue to direct the University of Arizona's Program in Integrative Medicine to lead a transformation in health care by educating and supporting a community of professionals expert in the principles and practice of this new system.

The Program in Integrative Medicine seeks to achieve its goal through four strategies:

1. *Training.* The Program prepares physicians to be practitioners and exemplars of integrative medicine, and leaders of programs and institutions across the country. Academic health centers, hospitals, and managed-care firms routinely seek physicians trained at the Program in Integrative Medicine for staff and leadership positions. Training is offered to physicians, nurse practitioners, residents, medical students, and others in both residential and distance-learning settings.

2. *National initiative.* The Program develops physician leadership across the country, provides curricular materials, prepares papers for medical publications, and helps to ensure the participation of integrative medicine physicians in national policy making.

3. *Research.* Investigators show a skeptical medical community how complex integrative-treatment approaches can be evaluated at a high

level of rigor without reducing them to single interventions isolated from other factors of body, mind, and spirit. Since 2002, the Program has received more than $3 million from the NIH and other sources for research and the training of researchers in integrative medicine.

4. *Clinical care.* More than three thousand persons have received treatment at the Program's outpatient clinic, and the waiting list is long.

For more information, visit *www.integrativemedicine.arizona.edu*

Notes

1. IMMORTALITY

13 Until 1961, researchers believed: L. Hayflick and P. S. Moorhead, "The Limited *In Vitro* Lifetime of Human Diploid Cell Strains," *Experimental Aging Research* 25 (1961), pp. 585–621.

14 HeLa cells, however, can divide indefinitely: Leonard Hayflick, *How and Why We Age* (New York: Ballantine, 1996), p. 115.

16 But that is another story: Rebecca Skloot, "Henrietta's Dance," *Johns Hopkins University Magazine,* April 2000; Beth Potier, "Filmmaker Immortalizes 'Immortal' Cells," *Harvard University Gazette,* July 19, 2001.

17 In 1985, Drs. Carol Greider and Elizabeth Blackburn: C. W. Greider and E. H. Blackburn, "Identification of a Specific Telomere Terminal Transferase Activity in *Tetrahymena* Extracts," *Cell* 43 (1985), pp. 405–13.

18 Examples are embryonic stem cells, . . . adult stem cells, . . . and germ cells: Stem Cell Information: The Official National Institutes of Health Resource for Stem Cell Research, http://stemcells.nih.gov/.

21 I have written elsewhere: Andrew Weil, M.D., *Spontaneous Healing: How to Discover and Enhance Your Body's Natural Ability to Maintain and Heal Itself* (New York: Ballantine, 1996), p. 81.

22 This has been successful with human fibroblasts: F. S. Wyllie et al., "Telomerase Prevents the Accelerated Cell Ageing of Werner Syndrome Fibroblasts," *Nature Genetics* 24, no. 1 (January 2000), pp. 16–17.

24 **Olshansky is the coauthor (with Bruce A. Carnes):** S. Jay Olshansky and Bruce A. Carnes, *The Quest for Immortality: Science at the Frontiers of Aging* (New York: W. W. Norton, 2001).

24 **"Position Statement on Human Aging":** S. Jay Olshansky, Leonard Hayflick, and Bruce A. Carnes, "Position Statement on Human Aging," *Journals of Gerontology A: Biological Sciences and Medical Sciences* 57 (2002), pp. 292–97.

26 **But nature has strongly favored the sexual method:** Olshansky and Carnes, *The Quest for Immortality,* pp. 50–79.

28 **Olshansky and Carnes write:** ibid., p. 52.

29 **One theory of aging postulates accumulated errors in the DNA:** Alexander P. Spence, *Biology of Human Aging,* 2nd ed. (Upper Saddle River, N.J.: Prentice Hall, 1999), pp. 21–22.

29 **Thomas Perls, M.D., who has studied the genetics of longevity:** Thomas Perls, M.D., personal communication, 2004.

31 **A favorite novel of mine that touches on this theme is *The Sibyl*:** Pär Lagerkvist, *The Sibyl,* translated by Naomi Walford (New York: Vintage, 1963), pp. 12, 17–18.

2. SHANGRI-LAS AND FOUNTAINS OF YOUTH

35 **"Never had Shangri-La offered more concentrated loveliness":** James Hilton, *Lost Horizon* (New York: Pocket Books, 1960), p. 160.

35 **They call these the *antediluvian, hyperborean,* and *fountain* legends:** Olshansky and Carnes, *The Quest for Immortality,* pp. 44–49.

36 **There is no scientific evidence for greater longevity in any past age:** ibid., pp. 70–72.

36 **This occurs to Conway:** Hilton, *Lost Horizon,* p. 70.

37 **The secret ingredient:** ibid., p. 136.

37 **Father Perrault:** ibid., p. 140.

37 **In every case, the claims turned out to be unsubstantiated:** Hayflick, *How and Why We Age,* pp. 196–202.

38 **a summary of the MacArthur Foundation Study of Aging in America:** John W. Rowe and Robert L. Kahn, *Successful Aging* (New York: Pantheon, 1998).

39 **Studies of centenarians have become more common:** The New England Centenarian Study, www.bumc.bu.edu/Dept/Home.aspx?DepartmentID=361; The Okinawa Centenarian Study, www.okinawaprogram.com; The Georgia Centenarian Study, www.geron.uga.edu/research/centenarianstudy.php.

39 **Leonard W. Poon:** Judy Purdy, "Hale and Hearty at 100," *University of Georgia Research Reporter* 25, no. 1 (Summer 1995).

40 **It is Okinawa:** Bradley J. Willcox, D. Craig Willcox, and Makoto Suzuki, *The Okinawa Program: How the World's Longest Lived People Achieve Everlasting Health—And How You Can Too* (New York: Clarkson Potter, 2001).

41 **Bitter melon:** A. Raman and C. Lau, "Anti-diabetic Properties and Phytochemistry of *Momordica charantia* L. (Cucurbitaceae)," *Phytomedicine* 2, no. 4 (1996) pp. 349–62.

42 **Turmeric:** http://new-chapter.com/research/turmeric.html.

43 **"In Okinawa there are none of the age-guessing games . . .":** Willcox, Willcox, and Makoto, *The Okinawa Program*, p. 5.

45 **[*Kajimaya*] . . . is arranged by the community:** ibid., p. 231.

46 **Okinawan longevity is now beginning to diminish:** Norimitsu Onishi, "On U.S. Fast Food, Okinawans Are Super-Sized," *New York Times,* March 30, 2004, p. A-1.

48 **I have written elsewhere about ginseng:** Weil, *Spontaneous Healing,* pp. 179–80; Andrew Weil, M.D., *8 Weeks to Optimum Health: A Proven Program for Taking Full Advantage of Your Body's Natural Healing Power* (New York: Ballantine, 1998), pp. 130–32, 136–37.

48 **Reishi:** Terry Willard, *Reishi Mushroom: Herb of Spiritual Potency and Medical Wonder* (Issaquah, Wash.: Sylvan Press, 1991); S. Wachtel-Galor, B. Tomlinson, and I. F. F. Benzie, "*Ganoderma lucidum* (Lingzhi), A Chinese Medicinal Mushroom: Biomarker Responses in a Controlled Human Supplementation Study," *British Journal of Nutrition* 91, no. 2 (2004), pp. 263–69.

50 **arctic root:** Richard P. Brown, Patricia L. Gerbarg, and Barbara Graham, *The Rhodiola Revolution: Transform Your Health with the Herbal Breakthrough of the 21st Century* (Emmaus, Pa.: Rodale Press, 2004); R. P. Brown, P. L. Gerbarg, and

Z. Ramazanov, "*Rhodiola rosea:* A Phytomedicinal Overview," *HerbalGram* 56 (2002), pp. 40–52.

50 **many other natural products are known as tonics or adaptogens:** I. I. Brekhman and I. V. Dardymov, "New Substances of Plant Origin Which Increase Non-Specific Resistance," *Annual Review of Pharmacology* 9 (1968), pp. 419–30.

51 **The best candidate in this group is human growth hormone (HGH):** Roy G. Smith and Michael O. Thorner, *Human Growth Hormone: Research and Clinical Practice* (Totowa, N.J.: Humana Press, 2000).

53 **an article by Dr. Daniel Rudman:** D. Rudman et al., "Effects of Human Growth Hormone in Men over 60 Years Old," *New England Journal of Medicine* 323, no. 1 (1990), pp. 1–6.

56 **Seymour (Si) Reichlin:** personal communication, 2004.

3. ANTIAGING MEDICINE

60 **The Taoists equated this with emissions of semen:** Eric Yudelove and Eric Steven Yudelove, *Taoist Yoga and Sexual Energy: Internal Alchemy and Chi Kung* (St. Paul, Minn.: Llewellyn, 2000).

60 **"Curiously, breathing the air of young virgin boys . . .":** Olshansky and Carnes, *The Quest for Immortality,* p. 41.

60 *The Joy of Laziness:* Peter Axt and Michaela Axt-Gadermann, *The Joy of Laziness: Why Life Is Better Slower—And How to Get There* (Alameda, Calif.: Hunter House, 2003).

60 **"cellular therapy":** Robert Thomson, "Niehans Cellular Therapy," *Grosset Encyclopedia of Natural Medicine* (New York: Grosset & Dunlap, 1980).

62 **"It is important to note that those who practice 'orthodox' medicine . . .":** www.extendlife.com/livecell.html.

63 **the American Academy of Anti-Aging Medicine:** www.world health.net.

63 **"Position Statement on Human Aging":** Olshansky, Hayflick, and Carnes, "Position Statement on Human Aging."

63 **Here is a representative quote from that article:** S. J. Olshansky, L. Hayflick, and B. A. Carnes, "No Truth to the Fountain of Youth," *Scientific American* 14, no. 3 (2002), pp. 98–102.

64 **Dr. Klatz sent an "Urgent Message":** http://www.anti-aging-secrets.info/antiagingarticles/issue24.html.

69 **In fact, the latter approach, known as "compression of morbidity":** J. F. Fries, "Aging, Illness, and Health Policy: Implications of the Compression of Morbidity," *Perspectives in Biological Medicine* 3, no. 31 (1988), pp. 407–28.

72 **"There are no death or aging genes—period":** Stephen S. Hall, *Merchants of Immortality: Chasing the Dream of Human Life Extension* (Boston: Houghton Mifflin, 2003), p. 203.

72 **"There are no genes for aging. I'll say that categorically":** ibid., p. 9.

72 **Perls and his colleagues identified a region on human chromosome 4:** A. A. Puca et al., "A Genome-Wide Scan for Linkage to Human Exceptional Longevity Identifies a Locus on Chromosome 4," *Proceedings of the National Academy of Sciences* 98, no. 18 (2001), pp. 10505–10508.

72 **(Some longevity genes might affect the transport of cholesterol . . .):** N. Barzilai et al., "Unique Lipoprotein Phenotype and Genotype Associated with Exceptional Longevity," *Journal of the American Medical Association* 290 (2003), pp. 2030–40.

72 **Michael Rose, an evolutionary biologist:** M. R. Rose, "Genetics of Increased Lifespan in *Drosophila*," *Bioessays* 11 (1989), pp. 132–35.

73 **"caloric restriction with adequate nutrition":** Hayflick, *How and Why We Age,* pp. 284–95; www.infoaging.org (search "caloric restriction").

73 **advocates of caloric restriction have published life-extension diet plans:** Brian Delaney and Lisa Walford, *The CR Diet: A Practical Guide to Living 120 Vital Years* (New York: Marlowe, 2004).

74 **Caloric restriction is a form of stress for an organism:** Hayflick, *How and Why We Age.*

74 **Some of the most provocative work has involved a species of nematode:** C. J. Kenyon et al., "A *C. elegans* Mutant That Lives Twice as Long as Wild Type," *Nature* 366 (1993), pp. 461–64.

75 **Kenyon has also recently cofounded a company:** Elixir Pharmaceuticals, www.elixirpharm.com.

75 **Cynthia Kenyon replied:** D. E. Duncan, "The Biologist Who Extends Lifespans," *Discover* 25, no. 3 (March 2004), pp. 16–19.

76 **They found a promising candidate in resveratrol:** Nicholas Wade, "Study Spurs Hope of Finding Way to Increase Human Life," *New York Times,* August 25, 2003; K. T. Howitz et al., "Small Molecule Activators of Sirtuns Extend *Saccharomyces cerevisiae* Lifespan," *Nature* 425 (September 11, 2003), pp. 191–96.

77 **Longevinex:** www.longevinex.com.

78 **Fernando Torres-Gil:** "The Boomers Are Coming: Challenges of Aging in the New Millennium," testimony before the Special Committee on Aging of the United States Senate, November 8, 1999, serial number 106–20 (Washington, D.C.: U.S. Government Printing Office, 2000); F. Torres-Gil, "Toward a New Politics of Aging in America," *In Depth: A Journal for Values and Public Policy* 2, no. 3 (1992), pp. 37–38.

79 **These are just a few of the concerns facing a society:** H. J. Aron and W. B. Schwartz, *Coping with Methuselah: The Impact of Molecular Biology on Medicine and Society* (Washington, D.C.: Brookings Institution Press, 2004).

79 **A recent article by Susan Dominus:** "Life in the Age of Old, Old Age," *New York Times Magazine,* February 22, 2004, p. 24.

4. WHY WE AGE

82 **"Aging is a deteriorative process":** Leonard Hayflick, quoted in Hall, *Merchants of Immortality,* p. 10.

83 **"Caramelization occurs in a sequence of six steps":** www.agsci.ubc.ca/courses/fnh/410/colour/3_81.htm.

83 **It is called the Maillard reaction:** J. O'Brien, H. E. Nursten, M. J. C. Crabbe, and J. M. Ames, *The Maillard Reaction in Foods and Medicine* (London: Royal Society of Chemistry, 1998). See also Harold McGee, *On Food and Cooking: The Science and Lore of the Kitchen* (New York: Scribner's, 2004), pp. 778–79.

84 **"The implications of these facts . . .":** Peter Forbes, "Recipe for Success," *Guardian,* January 23, 2003.

85 **Dr. Anthony Cerami:** A. Cerami, H. Vlassara, and M. Brownlee, "Hypothesis: Glucose as a Mediator of Aging," *Journal of the American Geriatric Society* 33, no. 9 (1985), pp. 626–34.

85 **Cross-linked proteins in the brain:** L. Melton, "AGE Breakers," *Scientific American,* July 2000, p. 16; L. Lorand,

"Neurodegenerative Diseases and Transglutaminase," *Proceedings of the National Academy of Sciences* 93 (1996), pp. 14310–13.

86 cross-link breakers: A. Cerami, "Pharmaceutical Intervention of Advanced Glycation End Products," *Novartis Bulletin,* Symposium 235 (2000).

86 pimagedine: www.alteonpharma.com/pimag1.htm.

87 "thrifty genes": J. V. Neel, "Diabetes Mellitus: A 'Thrifty' Genotype Rendered Detrimental by 'Progress'?" *American Journal of Human Genetics* 14 (1962), pp. 353–62.

90 Lipofuscin is not one substance: U. T. Brunk and A. Terman, "Lipofuscin: Mechanisms of Age-Related Accumulation and Influence on Cell Function," *Free Radical Biology & Medicine* 33, no. 5 (2002), pp. 611–19.

91 the free radical theory of aging: Leonard Hayflick, *How and Why We Age,* pp. 244–48.

97 Here are the arguments against taking these supplements: Nick Lane, *Oxygen: The Molecule That Made the World* (New York: Oxford University Press, 2002), Chap. 9.

98 Later research showed that smokers and ex-smokers: The Alpha-Tocopherol, Beta-Carotene Cancer Prevention Study Group, "The Effect of Vitamin E and Beta-carotene on the Incidence of Lung Cancer and Other Cancers in Male Smokers," *New England Journal of Medicine* 330 (1994), pp. 1029–35; G. E. Goodman et al., "The Beta-carotene and Retinol Efficacy Trial: Incidence of Lung Cancer and Cardiovascular Disease Mortality During 6-Year Follow-up after Stopping Beta-carotene and Retinol Supplements," *Journal of the National Cancer Institute* 96, no. 23 (2004), pp. 1743–50.

102 prolonged inflammation may be a common root of many chronic, degenerative diseases: T. Esch and G. B. Stefano, "Proinflammation: A Common Denominator or Initiator of Different Pathophysiological Disease Processes," *Medicine Science Monitor* 8, no. 5 (2002): HY1–9.

102 "Because oxidative stress is pivotal to our recovery from infections . . . .": Lane, *Oxygen,* pp. 296–301.

103 The Grenville Mountains: http://www.lithoprobe.ca/media/slideset/slides/growth16.asp.

105 **We are subject to the Second Law of Thermodynamics:** Hayflick, *How and Why We Age,* pp. 257–58; Harold Blum, *Time's Arrow and Evolution* (Princeton, N.J.: Princeton University Press, 1968).

5. THE DENIAL OF AGING

109 **In April 2003, the EPA proposed reducing the value:** Don Hopey, "What's an Older Person's Life Worth?" *Pittsburgh Post-Gazette,* April 15, 2003.

111 **Here is an excerpt from a *New York Times* article:** Ginia Bellafante, "Is This Cream Worth $500?" *New York Times,* June 15, 2003, Section 9, p. 1.

113 **diosgenin:** www.ibiblio.org/herbmed/archives/Best/1995/yam. html.

113 **IGF is a known tumor promoter:** V. A. Blakesley et al., "Role of the IGF-1 Receptor in Mutagenesis and Tumor Promotion," *Journal of Endocrinology* 152 (1997), pp. 339–44.

114 **More than 70 percent of those who opt for cosmetic surgery:** See the Web site of the American Society of Plastic Surgeons, www.plasticsurgery.org.

115 **In the words of a female plastic surgeon:** Daphne Merkin, "Keeping the Forces of Decrepitude at Bay," *New York Times,* May 2, 2004, Style section.

115 **I agree with Carl Jung, who wrote:** C. J. Jung, *Man in Search of a Soul* (New York: Harcourt Brace, 1936), p. 129.

115 **"How is it really":** Merkin, "Keeping the Forces of Decrepitude at Bay."

115 **"Aging is nature's way of preparing us for death":** ibid.

116 **"I suppose the one good thing":** ibid.

120 **But Oscar Wilde gave this advice:** quoted ibid.

6. THE VALUE OF AGING

125 **Consider this description of Old Rip Van Winkle's twelve-year-old Special Reserve:** www.missionliquor.com/Store/Qstore/Qstore.cgi (search "Van Winkle").

125 **"My family has always believed . . .":** www.Cocktailtimes.com/ distillery/ky/4.aging.shtml.

125 "Old whiskey is just more interesting . . .": Julian Van Winkle III, personal communication, 2004.

128 One authority describes it: www.bbr.com.

129 Here is what Château d'Yquem's Web site has to say: www.chateau-Yquem.com.

130 "milk's leap toward immortality": Clifton Fadiman (1904–99), American radio host, author, and editor.

132 I read an article in *The New Yorker*: Burkhard Bilger, "Raw Faith," *The New Yorker*, August 19 and 26, 2003.

133 The Abbey of Regina Laudis: Sara Davidson, "What They Did for Bliss," *O Magazine*, March 2004 (available at www.saradavidson.com); see also www.abbeyofreginalaudis.com.

135 "Beef, like fine wine, improves with age": www.beefinfo.org/aging.cfm.

136 "Still no one denies that dry aging . . .": Richard Chamberlain of Chamberlain's Steak & Chop House, Dallas, Texas, quoted in "Almost Everything You Need to Know About Dry Aged Beef," www.askthemeatman.com/dry_aging_beef_info.htm.

136 Jeffrey Steingarten, has this to say: Jeffrey Steingarten, *It Must Have Been Something I Ate* (New York: Alfred A. Knopf, 2002), pp. 460–61.

137 The Jomon Cedar: Thomas Pakenham, *Remarkable Trees of the World* (New York: W. W. Norton, 2002), pp. 50–51.

137 *Lord of the Rings*: J. R. R. Tolkien, *The Two Towers: Being the Second Part of the Lord of the Rings* (Boston: Houghton Mifflin, 1993), pp. 66ff.

138 the venerable Tule Tree of southern Mexico: Pakenham, *Remarkable Trees of the World*, pp. 24–29.

139 Bonsai: www.bonsaisite.com.

140 The bristlecone pines: Pakenham, *Remarkable Trees of the World*, pp. 71–77; also www.sonic.net/bristlecone/growth.html.

140 Here is Leonard Hayflick on the subject: Hayflick, *How and Why We Age*, p. 35.

142 At the end of the nineteenth century: Richard Ward, personal communication, 2004.

144 A Tucson couple named Ted and Virginia: Dennis Gaffney, "A Hand-Woven Treasure," www.pbs.org/wgbh/pages/roadshow/series/highlights/2002/tucson/tucson_follow1.html.

146 **the influenza pandemic of 1918 in Philadelphia:** John M. Barry,
*The Great Influenza: The Epic Story of the Deadliest Plague in
History* (New York: Penguin, 2004), pp. 197–227.

8. BODY I: THE OUNCE OF PREVENTION

158 **the sequencing of the human genome:** For information on the
Human Genome Project, see www.genome.gov.

158 **Studies of monozygotic (identical) twins:** Jeff Wheelwright,
"Study the Clones First," *Discover* 25, no. 8 (August 2004).

159 For more information on diet and breast cancer, see
http://envirocancer.cornell.edu/link/diet/link.diet.cfm.

161 **(It does not do so in "primitive" tribal cultures.):** Marshall David
Sahlins, *Stone Age Economics* (Chicago: Aldine, 1972).

162 **"fractionated cholesterol screening":** H. Robert Superko (with
Laura Tucker), *Before the Heart Attacks: A Revolutionary
Approach to Detecting, Preventing, and Even Reversing Heart
Disease* (Emmaus, Pa.: Rodale Press, 2003).

162 **electron beam computerized tomography (EBCT):** "American
College of Cardiology/American Heart Association Expert
Consensus Document on Electron-Beam Computed Tomography
for the Diagnosis and Prognosis of Coronary Artery Disease,"
Journal of the American College of Cardiology 36 (2000),
pp. 326–40.

168 **It is quite possible that our criteria for obesity:** Paul Campos, *The
Obesity Myth: Why America's Obsession with Weight Is
Hazardous to Your Health* (New York: Gotham, 2004).

168 **Here I will note that those who are somewhat overweight in
middle age:** ibid.

9. BODY II: THE ANTI-INFLAMMATORY DIET

174 **Asthma is increasing in frequency all over the world, for reasons
that are not clear:** A. J. Woolcock and J. K. Peat, "Evidence for the
Increase in Asthma Worldwide," *CIBA Foundation Symposia* 206
(1997), pp. 122–39, 157–59.

174 **The consensus among cardiologists today is that inflammation:**
J. Danesh, P. Whincup, M. Walker et al., "Low Grade

Inflammation and Coronary Heart Disease: Prospective Study and Updated Meta-Analysis," *British Medical Journal* 321 (2000), pp. 199–204.

175 **One neurologist who specializes:** David Perlmutter, *Brain Recovery.com: Powerful Therapy for Challenging Brain Disorders* (Naples, Fla.: Perlmutter Health Center, 2000).

175 **New research suggests that microinflammation:** G. Barbara et al., "A Role for Inflammation in Irritable Bowel Syndrome?" *Gut* 51 (2002), pp. 141–44.

178 **Sir John Vane:** See http://nobelprize.org/medicine/laureates/1982/.

178 **Many authorities on nutrition believe that the ratio of omega-6 to omega-3 fatty acids:** Andrew Weil, M.D., *Eating Well for Optimum Health: The Essential Guide to Bringing Health and Pleasure Back to Eating* (New York: Quill, 2001); Walter C. Willett and P. J. Skerrett, *Eat, Drink, and Be Healthy: The Harvard Medical School Guide to Healthy Eating* (New York: Free Press, 2002); Artemis P. Simopoulos and Jo Robinson, *The Omega Diet: The Lifesaving Nutritional Program Based on the Diet of the Island of Crete* (New York: HarperPerennial, 1999).

182 **AGEs can directly promote inflammation:** R. C. de Groof, "Remodeling of Age- and Diabetes-Related Changes in Extracellular Matrix," *Proceedings of 10th International Association of Biomedical Gerontology* (New York: New York Academy of Sciences, 2003).

188 **Dr. David Heber:** *What Color Is Your Diet?* (New York: Regan, 2002).

189 **anthocyanins:** "Special Issue on Anthocyanins—More than Nature's Colours," *Journal of Biomedicine and Biotechnology* 2004, no. 5 (December 1, 2004).

190 **Organically grown fruits and vegetables:** D. K. Asami et al., "Comparison of the Total Phenolic and Ascorbic Acid Content of Freeze-Dried and Air-Dried Marionberry, Strawberry, and Corn Grown Using Conventional, Organic, and Sustainable Agricultural Practices," *Journal of Agriculture and Food Chemistry* 51, no. 5 (2003), pp. 1237–41.

190 **In a preface to the program:** Izabela Konczak and Wei Zhang, "Anthocyanins—More than Nature's Colours," *Journal of Biomedicine and Biotechnology* 2004, no. 5 (December 1, 2004), p. 239.

192 **All true tea:** See www.teahealth.co.uk.

194 **Carotenoids:** H. Pfander, "Carotenoids: An Overview," *Methods in Enzymology* 213 (1992), pp. 3–13; H. Nishino, "Cancer Prevention by Carotenoids," *Mutation Research* 402 (1998), pp. 159–63. See also www.astaxanthin.org/carotenoids.htm.

195 **other health-protective compounds in plants:** See www.barc.usda.gov/bhnrc/pl/.

196 **compounds in plants we eat can actually modify the expression of our genes:** Anne Underwood and Jerry Adler, "Diet and Genes," *Newsweek,* January 17, 2005.

10. BODY III: SUPPLEMENTS

197 **Now they say they are dangerous:** "CR Investigates: Dangerous Supplements Still at Large," *Consumer Reports* 69, no. 5 (May 2004), p. 12.

198 **For example, nature produces vitamin E in a complex:** M. G. Traber and L. Packer, "Vitamin E: Beyond Antioxidant Function," *American Journal of Clinical Nutrition* 62 (1995), pp. 1501S–1509S. See also http://ods.od.nih.gov/factsheets/vitamine.asp.

198 **Beta-carotene by itself can actually increase cancer risks:** See citations for p. 79 above.

199 **indole-3-carbinol:** C. M. Cover et al., "Indole-3-carbinol Inhibits the Expression of Cyclin-dependent Kinase-6 and Induces a G1 Cell Cycle Arrest of Human Breast Cancer Cells Independent of Estrogen Receptor Signalling," *Journal of Biological Chemistry* 273, no. 7 (1998), pp. 3838–47.

201 **Ames investigated two dietary supplements in rats:** T. N. Hagen et al., "Feeding Acetyl-L-carnitine and Lipoic Acid to Old Rats Significantly Improves Metabolic Function While Decreasing Oxidative Stress," *Proceedings of the National Academy of Sciences* 99, no. 4 (2002), pp. 1870–75.

201 **Juvenon:** See www.juvenon.com.

201 **In August 2003 the *Berkeley Wellness Letter:*** See "Wellness Guide to Dietary Supplements: The Latest on ALA." www.berkeley wellness.com/html/ds/dsAlphaLipoicAcid.php.

204 *Co-Q-10:* Go to www.cancer.gov and search for "Coenzyme Q PDQ."

205 **proanthocyanidins, or PCOs:** Michael Murray and Joseph
Pizzorno, eds., *The Textbook of Natural Medicine,* 2nd ed.
(London: Churchill Livingston, 1999), pp. 899–902.

205 *Alpha-lipoic acid:* See www.lef.org/abstracts/codex/alpha_lipoic_
acid_abstracts.htm (Search "Ames" to find papers by Bruce Ames).

206 *Ginger and turmeric:* For ginger, see Mark Blumenthal et al., eds.,
The ABC Clinical Guide to Herbs (Austin, Tex.: American
Botanical Council, 2003), pp. 171–83. For turmeric, see
www.new-chapter.com.

207 *Aspirin:* Diar Muid Jeffreys, *Aspirin: The Remarkable Story of a
Wonder Drug* (New York: Bloomsbury USA, 2004). See also
www.aspirin-foundation.com/uses/cancer.html.

208 **ibuprofen:** www.nlm.nih.gov/medlineplus/print/druginfo/
medmaster/a682159.html.

208 DHEA: *The Medical Letter* 47, no. 1208 (May 9, 2005),
pp. 37–38.

210 *Astragalus:* Dennis J. McKenna, Kenneth Jones, Kerry Hughes,
and Sheila Humphrey, *Botanical Medicines: The Desk Reference
for Major Herbal Supplements,* 2nd ed. (New York: Haworth
Herbal Press, 2002), pp. 1–17.

211 *Immune-enhancing mushrooms:* Christopher Hobbs and Harriet
Beinfield, *Medicinal Mushrooms: An Exploration of Tradition,
Healing & Culture* (Santa Cruz, Calif.: Botanica Press, 2003). See
also www.fungi.com.

212 **Milk thistle:** McKenna et al., *Botanical Medicines,* pp. 765–808.

213 *Ginseng:* ibid., pp. 505–47.

213 *Eleuthero ginseng:* ibid., pp. 255–71.

213 *Arctic root:* See reference for p. 40 above.

214 *Cordyceps:* McKenna et al., *Botanical Medicines,* pp. 169–84.

214 **Marcus Tullius Cicero . . . wrote:** *De Senectute,* translated by
E. S. Shuckburgh; the full text is given at http://ancienthistory.
about.com/library/bl/bl_text_cicero_desenec.htm.

215 *Testosterone:* Catharyn T. Liverman, Dan G. Blazer, and the
National Research Council, *Testosterone and Aging: Clinical
Research Directions* (Washington, D.C.: National Academies
Press, 2004). See also www.mayoclinic.com/invoke.cfm?id=
MC00030.

215 *Ashwagandha:* See www.herbmed.org/Herbs/Herb136.htm.

11. BODY IV: PHYSICAL ACTIVITY

217 **MacArthur Foundation's Study of Aging in America:** John W. Rowe and Robert L. Kahn, *Successful Aging* (New York: Pantheon, 1998), pp. 97–111.

217 **Here is a description of one:** Anthony Faiola, "Old but Not Retiring: Japan's Astoundingly Healthy Seniors Climb Peaks, Cross Deserts, Sail Seas," *Washington Post,* October 10, 2004, p. A-1.

220 **Repeated concussive injuries, as in football and soccer:** Barry Yeoman, "Lights Out: Can Contact Sports Lower Your Intelligence?" *Discover* 25, no. 12 (December 2004).

220 **Perhaps this is the reason that ALS . . . appears more frequently in athletes:** N. Scarmeas et al., "Premorbid Weight, Body Mass, and Varsity Athletics in ALS," *Neurology* 59 (2002), pp. 773–75.

230 **It can even improve the physical and mental well-being of old people:** Wayne Westcott et al., "Strength Training Elderly Nursing Home Patients," *Mature Fitness* (formerly *Senior Fitness Bulletin*) 6, no. 4 (1999), available online at www.seniorfitness.net/strength.htm.

231 **Pilates method:** www.pilatesmethodalliance.org.

232 **yoga:** Rodney Yee, *Moving Toward Balance: 8 Weeks of Yoga with Rodney Yee* (Emmaus, Pa.: Rodale Press, 2004).

233 **older people who practice tai chi are less likely to fall:** S. L. Wolf et al., "Intense Tai Chi Exercise Training and Fall Occurrences in Older, Transitionally Frail Adults: A Randomized Controlled Trial," *Journal of the American Geriatrics Society* 51, no. 12 (2003), pp. 1693–1701.

12. BODY V: REST AND SLEEP

237 **People who nap generally enjoy better mental health:** Scott S. Campbell et al., "Effects of a Nap on Nighttime Sleep and Waking Function in Older Subjects," *Journal of the American Geriatrics Society* 53, no. 1 (2005), p. 48.

238 **Anthropologists note that in "primitive" cultures:** See reference for p. 161 above.

241 **Dr. Rubin Naiman:** personal communication, 2005. See also www.drnaiman.com.

242 **The coming of night brought dangers:** A. Roger Ekirch, *At Day's Close: Night in Times Past* (New York: W. W. Norton, 2005).

243 **Both Dr. Naiman and I believe it's important to access that realm:** Andrew Weil, M.D., *The Marriage of the Sun and Moon: Dispatches from the Frontiers of Consciousness,* rev. ed. (Boston: Houghton Mifflin, 2004).

244 **Pay attention to sleep hygiene:** www.thesleepsite.com/hygiene.html. See also Andrew Weil, M.D., *Natural Health, Natural Medicine,* rev. ed. (Boston: Houghton Mifflin, 2004), Chap. 6.

245 **Melatonin:** www.ahrq.gov/clinic/epcsums/melatsum.htm.

13. BODY VI: TOUCH AND SEX

247 **Touch is a basic requirement:** Robert W. Hatfield, "Touch and Human Sexuality," in V. Bullough and A. Stein, eds., *Human Sexuality: An Encyclopedia* (New York: Garland Publishing, 1994).

248 **some research suggests that seniors who remain sexually active:** Warren E. Leary, "Older People Enjoy Sex, Survey Says," *New York Times,* September 29, 1998, p. F-8; Debora Demeter, "Sex and the Elderly," full text version available on www.umkc.edu/sites/hsw/age/.

250 **There are even Internet dating services for the elderly:** For example, www.SeniorMatch.com.

14. MIND I: STRESS

251 **Cortisol . . . is directly toxic to neurons:** Robert M. Sapolsky, *Why Zebras Don't Get Ulcers: An Updated Guide to Stress, Stress-Related Diseases, and Coping,* 2nd ed. (New York: W. H. Freeman, 1998).

252 **the "relaxation response":** Herbert Benson, *The Relaxation Response* (New York: HarperTorch, 1976).

253 **Recently, scientists demonstrated:** E. S. Epel et al., "Accelerated Telomere Shortening in Response to Life Stress," *Proceedings of*

the National Academy of Sciences 101, no. 49 (2004), pp. 17312–15.

15. MIND II: THOUGHTS, EMOTIONS, ATTITUDES

263 **Depression . . . can directly lower immunity:** L. McGuire et al., "Depressive Symptoms and Lymphocyte Proliferation in Older Adults," *Journal of Abnormal Psychology*, 111, no. 1 (2002).

263 **Cognitive behavioral therapy:** Judith S. Beck, *Cognitive Therapy: Basics and Beyond* (New York: Guilford Press, 1995).

264 **Five hundred years earlier, the Buddha taught:** Ron Leifer, *The Happiness Project: The Three Poisons That Cause the Suffering We Inflict on Ourselves and Others* (Ithaca, N.Y.: Snow Lion Publications, 1997).

264 **Moreover, these new forms of psychotherapy are effective:** See www.cognitivetherapy.com.

264 **Martin E. P. Seligman:** *Learned Optimism* (New York: Alfred A. Knopf, 1971).

266 ***Don't Think of an Elephant!:*** George Lakoff, *Don't Think of an Elephant!* (White River Junction, Vt.: Chelsea Green Publishing, 2004), p. 53.

269 **mindfulness-based stress reduction (MBSR):** See the Web site of the Center for Mindfulness in Medicine, Health Care, and Society (CFM) at www.umassmed.edu/cfm.

269 **Dr. Madan Kataria:** www.laughteryoga.org.

16. MIND III: MEMORY

272 **The central nervous system is highly plastic:** R. K. Carlin and P. Siekevitz, "Plasticity in the Central Nervous System: Do Synapses Divide?" *Proceedings of the National Academy of Sciences* 80, no. 11 (1983), pp. 3517–21.

273 **Nicotine affects brain chemistry in several ways:** Wanda Hamilton, "Nicotine Benefits," full text with references available at www.forces.org/evidence/hamilton/other/nicotine.htm. See also A. Ott et al., "Effect of Smoking on Global Cognitive Function in Nondemented Elderly," *Neurology* 62 (2004), pp. 920–24.

274 **Ginkgo . . . has been shown to slow the progression of dementia:**

P. L. LeBars et al., "A Placebo Controlled Double-Blind, Randomized Trial of an Extract of *Ginkgo biloba* for Dementia," *Journal of the American Medical Association* 278 (1997), pp. 1327–32.

275 **An objective group, the Alzheimer Research Forum, says:** www.alzforum.org/drg/drc/detail.asp?id=20.

275 *Phosphatidyl serine,* **or PS:** T. H. Crook et al., "Effects of Phosphatidylserine in Age-Associated Memory Impairment," *Neurology* 41, no. 5 (1991), pp. 644–49.

278 **A recent study reports that bilingual subjects:** E. Bialystock, "Bilingualism May Counter Effects of Aging," *Psychology and Aging* 19 (2004), pp. 290–303.

17. SPIRIT I: UNCHANGING ESSENCE

282 **Kathleen Dowling Singh:** "Taking a Spiritual Inventory," PBS television interview from *On Our Own Terms: Moyers on Dying,* 2000, transcript available at www.pbs.org/wnet/onourownterms/articles/inventory2.html.

284 **As Joseph Campbell wrote:** *The Hero with a Thousand Faces,* reprint ed. (Princeton, N.J.: Princeton University Press, 1972), pp. 56–57.

18. SPIRIT II: LEGACY

288 **I have looked over examples of this literature:** Harold Abrahams, ed., *Hebrew Ethical Wills* (Philadelphia: The Jewish Publication Society of America, 1926; facsimile edition, 1976).

290 **How interesting, then, that the ethical will is currently making a strong comeback:** Barry K. Baines, *Ethical Wills: Putting Your Values on Paper* (Cambridge, Mass.: Perseus Publishing, 2001); Barry K. Baines, *The Ethical Will Writing Guide Workbook* (Minneapolis: Josaba Ltd., 2001). See also www.ethicalwill.com.

Acknowledgments

The writing of this book required a great deal of research. I was fortunate to have the assistance of many persons in identifying, collecting, and evaluating relevant information, among them Dr. Howard Silverman, Dr. Seymour Reichlin, Dr. Jay Olshansky, Professor Fernando Gil-Torres, Dr. Rubin Naiman, and Dr. Victoria Maizes. I give special thanks to Sandra J. Wilmot and her editorial team at Rebus for preparing an excellent summary of research on the age pigment lipofuscin.

Persons who provided other material that went into these pages include Deborah Coryell, Adele Simmons, Kathy Goodman, Paul Stamets, Mother Noella Marcellino of the Abbey of Regina Laudis, Julian P. Van Winkle III of the Old Rip Van Winkle Distillery, and Richard Ward of Ifshin Violins.

I am grateful to my friends Tim McLean and Yoshiko Takaoka in Shizuoka, Japan, for introducing me to Okinawa and providing introductions and translation services there along with Remi Ie. Drs. Bradley and Craig Willcox also helped me meet people in those wonderful islands, as did Dr. David Itokazu and Mr. Hazama Yasuyuki of Ishigaki.

Several people read preliminary versions of the manuscript and made valuable suggestions for improving it, especially Kathy Goodman. I also thank Sara Davidson, Dr. Jim Nicolai, and Dr. Dan Shapiro.

My medical partner, Dr. Brian Becker, was the person responsible for fact-checking and gathering references. His services were first-rate and much appreciated.

On the home front, I had the wonderful assistance of Richard Baxter,

Karen Hill, and Dena Jaffee, as well as the always enjoyable company of Daisy and Jambo.

My editor at Alfred A. Knopf, Jonathan Segal, performed his usual magic in polishing the manuscript for publication. His help was always welcome. As ever, I am delighted to have the support of Sonny Mehta and of my agent, Richard Pine.

Vail, Arizona
February 2005

Index